CONTRAST AGENTS IN LIVER IMAGING

SERIES IN RADIOLOGY

VOLUME 25

*The titles published in this series are listed at the end of this volume.*

# CONTRASTAGENTS IN LIVER IMAGING

Edited by

DR. T. BALZER

*Clinical Development Diagnostics, Magnetic Resonance and Ultrasound Contrast Media, Schering AG, Berlin, Germany*

PROF. DR. B. HAMM

*Department of Radiology, Charité Hospital, Humboldt University, Schumannstr. 20/21, D-10098 Berlin, Germany*

and

DR. H.-P. NIENDORF

*Clinical Development Diagnostics, Magnetic Resonance and Ultrasound Contrast Media, Schering AG, Berlin, Germany*

SPRINGER-SCIENCE+BUSINESS MEDIA, B.V.

A catalogue record for this book is available from the British Library

ISBN 978-94-010-4213-0

**Library of Congress Cataloging-in-Publication Data**

Contrast agents in liver imaging / edited by Th. Balzer, B. Hamm and H.-P. Niendorf.
p. cm. — (Series in radiology; v. 25)
Includes index.
ISBN 978-94-010-4213-0 ISBN 978-94-011-0477-7 (eBook)
DOI 10.1007/978-94-011-0477-7
1. Liver—Imaging—Congresses. 2. Contrast media—Congresses.
I. Balzer, Th., II. Hamm, Bernd, Prof. Dr. III. Niendorf, H.- P.
IV. Series: Series in Radiolgy; 25.
[DNLM: 1. Liver Diseases—diagnosis—congresses. 2. Liver—pathology—congresses. 3. Diagnostic Imaging—methods—congresses. 4. Contrast Media—congresses. W1 SE719 v. 25 1995 / WI 700 C763 1995]
RC847.5.I42C66 1995
616.3'620754—dc20
DNLM/DLC 94-34131
for Library of Congresses CIP

**Copyright**



Typeset by EXPO Holdings, Malaysia.

# CONTENTS

# LIST OF CONTRIBUTORS

**T. BALZER**
Clinical Development Diagnostics
Magnetic Resonance and Ultrasound Contrast Media
Schering AG
Berlin
Germany

**M.E. BERNARDINO**
Department of Radiology
Emory University Hospital
1364 Clifton Road NE
Atlanta
GA 30322
USA

**F. BORCHARD**
Institut für Pathologie der Heinrich-Heine-Universität
Postfach 101007
D-40001 Düsseldorf
Germany

**S. DELORME**
Deutsches Krebsforschungszentrum
Forschungsschwerpunkt Radiologische Diagnostik und Therapie
Im Neuenheimer Feld 280
D-69120 Heidelberg
Germany

**P.C. FREENY**
Department of Radiology
University of Washington Medical Center
Seattle
WA 98034
USA

**J. GAA**
Department of Radiology
Massachusetts General Hospital
Harvard Medical School
Boston
MA 02114
USA

**B. HAMM**
Department of Radiology
Charité Hospital, Humboldt University
Schumannstr. 20/21
D-10098 Berlin
Germany

**G. MARCHAL**
Department of Radiology
University Hospitals
Herestraat 49
B-3000 Leuven
Belgium

**Y. NI**
Department of Radiology
University Hospitals
Herestraat 49
B-3000 Leuven
Belgium

**H.-P. NIENDORF**
Clinical Development Diagnostics
Magnetic Resonance and Ultrasound Contrast Media
Schering AG
Berlin
Germany

**R. PICHLMAYR**
Medizinische Hochschule Hannover
Klinik für Abdominal und Transplantationschirurgie
Konstanty-Gutschow-Str.8
D-30625 Hannover
Germany

**B. RINGE**
Georg-August-Universität
Abteilung Transplantationschirurgie
Robert-Koch-Str. 40
D-37075 Göttingen
Germany

**P.R. ROS**
Division of Abdominal Imaging and Magnetic Resonance Imaging
University of Florida College of Medicine
Gainesville
Florida
USA

**S. SAINI**
Department of Radiology
Massachusetts General Hospital
Harvard Medical School
Boston
MA 02114
USA

**U.P. SCHMIEDL**
Department of Radiology
University of Washington Medical Center
Seattle
WA 98034
USA
*currently working at:*
Diagnostic Imaging Sciences
University of Seattle

**G.T. SICA**
Department of Radiology
Brigham and Women's Hospital
75 Francis Street
Boston
MA 02115
USA

**M. TAUPITZ**
Department of Radiology
Charité Hospital
Humboldt University
Schumannstr. 20/21
D-10098 Berlin
Germany

**A. WEIMANN**
Medizinische Hochschule Hannover
Klinik für Abdominal und Transplantationschirurgie
Konstanty-Gutschow-Str.8
D-30625 Hannover
Germany

# INTRODUCTION

Recent advances in surgical procedures for the management of focal liver disease, ranging from an improved and extended resection strategy to the general availability of liver transplantation, have greatly increased the demand for diagnostic accuracy. Unfortunately, so far these demands have been only partially met by further technical developments such as colour-coded duplex sonography, spiral CT and marked improvements in magnetic resonance imaging. It is becoming increasingly clear that liver-specific contrast media are essential for utilizing these technical developments to their fullest advantage in patient care.

Against the background of diverse endeavours to develop such contrast media for all three imaging modalities, a workshop was held to explore the current methods of diagnostic imaging of the liver and to try to establish a profile for the future liver-specific contrast media.The idea behind the workshop was not only to allow radiologists from the various spheres to voice their opinions, but also to enter into an interdisciplinary discussion with both those who plan and perform therapies – particularly surgeons and internists – and those who are in a better position to judge the sensitivity and specificity of a method.

The chapters in this book are presented in the same order as the lectures. The pathologist's introductory and general overview is followed by other chapters on the individual imaging procedures such as ultrasound, CT and MRI, so that each of the three can be given the close attention it deserves.

All the authors and the discussion participants we were fortunate enough to engage have at least one thing in common – they are widely known within their disciplines for their outstanding scientific work. We would like to thank them again for giving up so much of their valuable time to participate in the workshop and for contributing so much to its success.

We are also indebted to the staff of Kluwer Academic Publishers for processing the manuscripts so expertly.

**Th. Balzer**
**B. Hamm**
**H.-P. Niendorf**

# 1

# FUNCTIONAL CYTOARCHITECTURE OF THE NORMAL LIVER AND FOCAL LIVER LESIONS

F. BORCHARD

## Introduction

The following paper focuses on two aspects of liver pathology, namely the presentation of functional cytoarchitecture of the liver relevant to the uptake or processing of contrast media and the description of the main focal liver lesions.

## Functional cytoarchitecture

The architecture of the liver is well known and has been studied by many methods, including transmission and scanning electron microscopy, immunohistochemistry and cell culture. In this paper, the functional role of various cell types in the normal and diseased liver will be elucidated.

Besides vascular components, connective tissue cells, nerves and a few inflammatory cells, there are seven main cell types in the liver, 3 of epithelial and 4 of sinusoidal origin (Table 1.1).

### *Epithelial cells*

The epithelial cells include hepatocytes, bile duct epithelia and oval cells. The functions of these cells are manifold and will not be reviewed in great detail. Hepatocytes show an expression of various plasma proteins, synthesis of cholesterol and bile, glyconeogenesis, glycolysis, and uptake of fatty acids. Bile duct epithelial cells form the lining of bile transport channels within the portal tracts and larger ducts. Oval cells are regenerative cells occurring in the periphery of the lobule after necrosis.

### *Mesenchymal cells*

These will be discussed in more detail.

**Table 1.1 Main cell types in the liver**

| |
|---|
| **Epithelial cells** |
| Hepatocytes |
| Bile duct epithelia |
| Small cells (oval, hepatoid, cholangioid) |
| **Sinusoidal cells** |
| Fenestrated endothelia |
| Kupffer cells (stellate cells) |
| Fat storing cells (Ito cells, lipocytes) |
| Pit cells |

### Fenestrated sinusoidal endothelia

The main component is the flat 'fenestrated' sinusoidal endothelial cell which has clusters of small pores in its cytoplasm; these pores, with a mean diameter of 100 nm (range 50–300 nm) are called sieve plates[1]. Although influenced by preparative methods, the size of the fenestrae may be influenced by a number of factors in vivo[1]. Fenestrated endothelial cells separate all liver sheets from the sinusoidal lumen (Figure 1.1) and constitute about 60% of the sinusoidal cells[2]. The fenestrated endothelia perform a number of functions as a graded barrier for exchange of fluid and particulate substances, clearance of macromolecules by endocytosis, removal of harmful pathogens, enzymes and collagen, as well as binding and uptake of lipoprotein. The fenestrated endothelial cells have receptors for hyaluronidase, chondroitin sulphate, mannose-terminated glycoprotein, Fc-fragment of IgG, and for lipopolysaccharide-binding proteins[3].

These fenestrated endothelia are unique in the human body and do not react with antibodies or lectins which stain ordinary, non-fenestrated endothelial cells (e.g. antibodies directed to CD 34 and F VIII-associated antigen, or UEA I-lectin). Such non-fenestrated endothelia occur in the vessels of the portal tract and within the central vein (Figure 1.2a).

The specialized fenestrated endothelia express the intercellular adhesion molecular ICAM 1 and are the

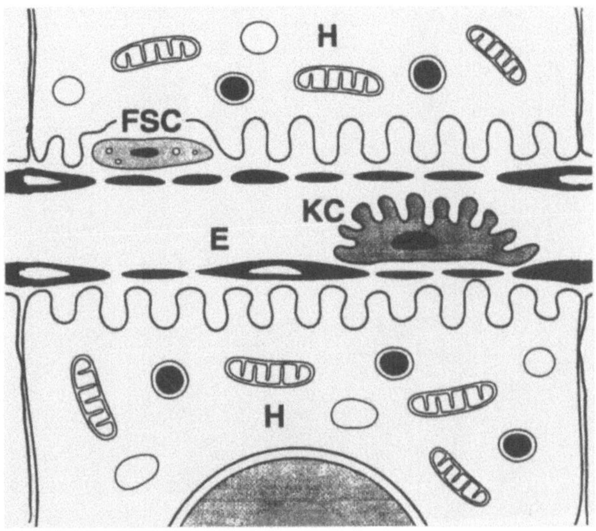


**Figure 1.1** The cellular composition of the sinusoidal wall. E = fenestrated endothelia, FSC = fat storing cell, KC = Kupffer cell

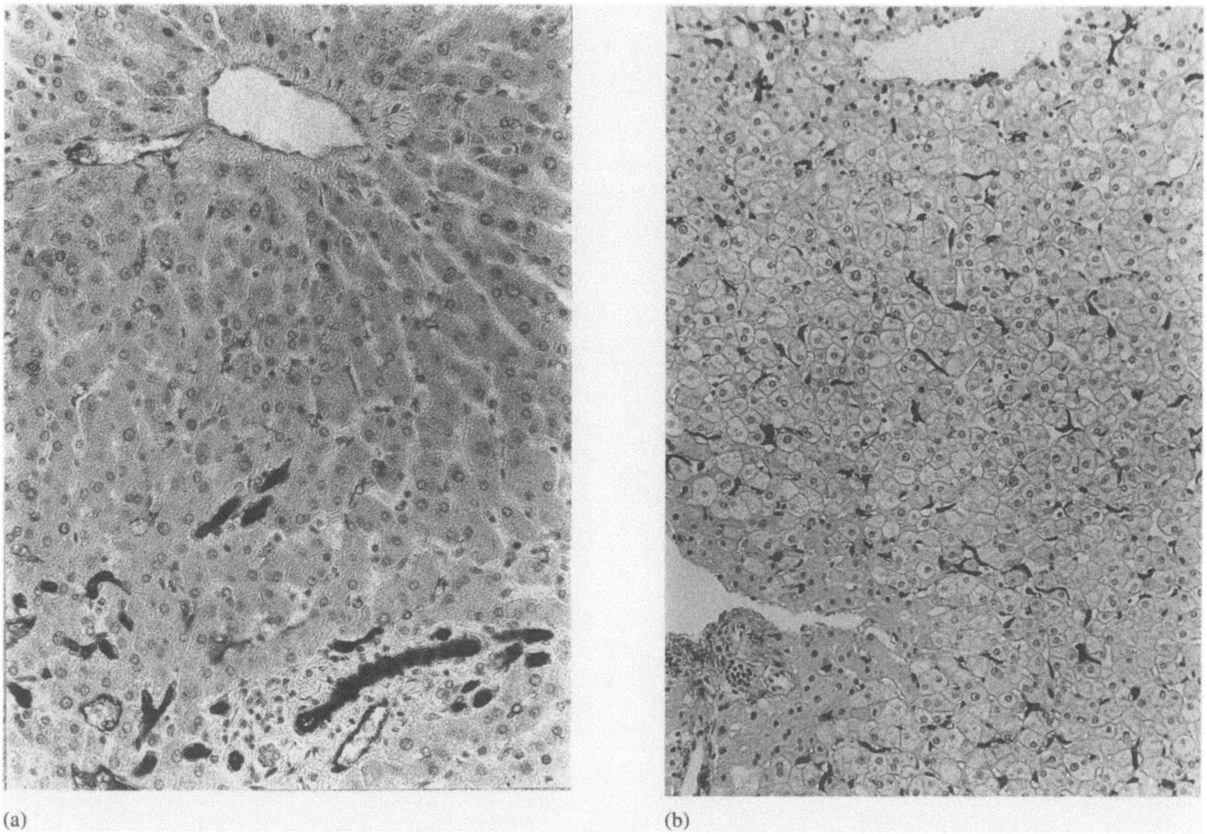

(a) (b)

**Figure 1.2** Immunohistochemistry of sinusoidal cells in the normal liver: (a) non-fenestrated endothelia (CD 34) in the portal tract and (b) even distribution of Kupffer-cells (PGM1) in the lobule. Avidin–Biotin, each 200×

prerequisite for the attachment of Kupffer cells. Thus the loss of fenestrated endothelia under pathological conditions usually also entails a loss of Kupffer cells (see below). In alcoholic liver disease[4] and in liver cirrhosis[5], there is loss of fenestrated endothelium (and Kupffer cells).

## Kupffer cells

Kupffer cells (stellate cells) are mobile macrophages, partly recruited from the bone marrow, that also have a small capacity to divide. They constitute about 31% of the sinusoidal cells of the liver[2]. Although a lobular gradient with a higher number in the periportal region has been described in the rat liver, by immunostaining, we found a fairly even distribution within the human liver lobule (Figure 1.2b). The Kupffer cells are mostly attached to the luminal surface of endothelial cells; they only rarely penetrate the endothelial coat and may contact the hepatocytes[2,6,7]. Like many other types of macrophages, they have various functions in two types of phagocytosis, either in receptor-mediated uptake of particulate matter or in non-receptor-dependent uptake of fluid or substances.

The macrophages can be immunohistochemically demonstrated by monoclonal antibodies that recognize normal histiocytes (e.g. PGM1, KP1/CD68 or Mac 387). The distribution of Kupffer cells depends on the presence of fenestrated endothelia so that a so-called ‘capillarization’ with non-fenestrated endothelia will lead to a loss of macrophages, e.g. in liver cirrhosis and hepatomas (see below).

## Fat storing cells

The fat storing cells (Ito cells) are situated underneath the fenestrated endothelial cells, within the space of Disse, and usually contain fat droplets and vitamin A. In liver damage, these cells may accumulate in centrilobular areas, transform into myofibroblasts and produce various types of collagen and laminin. Thus,

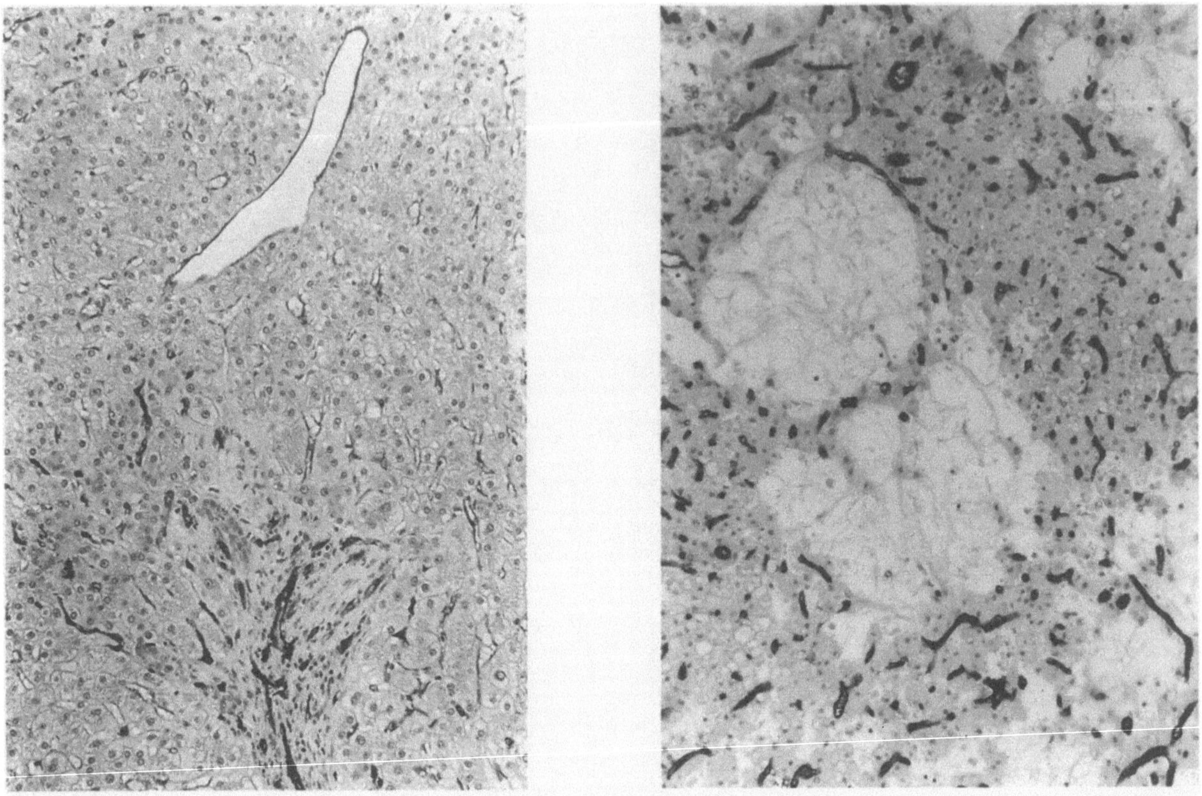

(a) (b)

**Figure 1.3** Immunohistochemical distribution of non-fenestrated endothelia (CD 34): (a) localization in the neighbourhood of fibrous septa in FNH and (b) 'capillarization' in liver cell adenoma with sparing in peliosis. Avidin–Biotin, each 200×

scarring of Disse spaces may occur, leading to a centrilobular fibrosis of meshwork type, e.g. in alcoholic hepatitis. Fat storing cells can be immunohistochemically detected by anti-smooth muscle antibodies. A modulation of intermediate filaments may occur in liver cirrhosis, where they also may express desmin[8].

Pit cells

The sparsely distributed pit cells were first thought to be endocrine cells because of their cytoplasmic granules, but have now been shown to be lymphocytes with natural killer activity.

## Focal liver lesions

### *Cysts*

The so-called 'cysts' comprise true cysts with an epithelial lining and pseudocysts which lack such a lining. Except for rare examples of (pseudo)-cystic neoplasias, liver cysts are mainly tumour-like lesions and occurred in about 0.4% in a series of abdominal ultrasonography[9]. The aetiology is either developmental or acquired: inflammatory, obstructive, traumatic, parasitic and neoplastic. The wall of congenital cysts is usually thin whereas the wall of acquired cysts is thicker. Among the truly non-neoplastic cysts, the solitary simple hepatic cysts are probably of mesothelial origin, whereas cysts in polycystic liver disease, intrahepatic bile duct cysts, congenital hepatic fibrosis and von Meyenburg complexes (microhamartoma) result from maldevelopment of bile ducts, sometimes accompanied by renal or pancreatic cysts[10]. The incidence of cystic bile ducts in autopsies has been stated as 0.15%[11]. Non-neoplastic cysts must be distinguished from rare cystadenoma and cystadenocarcinoma. Only the latter true neoplasms or symptomatic cysts should be treated.

### *Haemangioma*

Haemangiomas of the liver have an incidence of about 1% of autopsy cases, with a range of 0.4–20%[10]. However, in a meticulous legomedical study, haemangiomas with a mean size of 5.2 mm were seen in about 50% of a male population[12]. Since haemangiomas are more common in adults than in children, it has been postulated that not all of them are connatal hamartomas but that they may even arise in adults. Haemangiomas occur 4 times more frequently in adult women than in men, probably because female sexual hormones stimulate endothelial growth. Most haemangiomas lie in the subcapsular area. Haemangiomas with a diameter of more than 10 cm are called giant haemangiomas. Histologically, the cavernous type greatly outnumbers the rare capillary type. The blood-filled spaces are invested by an ordinary, non-fenestrated endothelium. There are no macrophages or intervening hepatocytes. Blood flow is usually low, thus causing the iris shutter phenomenon under radiological examination. The low blood flow may be the reason why central thrombi often develop, becoming organized and hyalinized. Haemangiomatosis is defined as a diffuse infiltration of liver tissue by differentiated capillaries. As complications in simple liver haemangiomas are rare, therapy is not indicated.

### *Focal nodular hyperplasia (FNH)*

The incidence of FNH in autopsy studies has been stated as 0.3%, representing about 2–8% of all primary liver tumours[10]. However, in a meticulous legomedical study of a male population[12], the incidence was 3.2% and the mean diameter was 0.8 cm. In up to 20% of the cases, multiple FNH can be seen. While earlier data suggested a major preponderance of FNH over adenomas, more recent data suggest a shift to adenomas so that the incidence of FNH is about twice that of adenoma. Clinically, FNH is a rare lesion and was seen in only 1 of 75 000 patients investigated by ultrasonography[13]. The ratio of male:female is 1:4. There is no correlation between the incidence of FNH and the use of contraceptives, but the latter may influence the size and multiplicity of the lesions and the occurrence of complications.

Macroscopically, the mean diameter in major series[14,15] was about 5–6 cm, with a range of 0.3–24 cm. Lesions of less than 5 cm are usually asymptomatic. In a meta analysis of 930 FNH, 57.7% were situated in the subcapsular area and 8.8% were pedunculated[16]. Although the margin of the lesions is sharp, they are not encapsulated. The majority of FNH have a central fibrous scar with radiating septae dividing the lesions into large nodes. The colour of the lesions is usually somewhat lighter than the surrounding hepatic tissue.

Microscopically, one of the hallmarks of FNH is a dysplastic artery within the central radiating scar. It is thought that the dysplastic artery is maldevelopmental in origin and that it leads to hepatocellular hyperplasia[17]. Pathogenetically, a massive increase of blood flow and focal thrombosis (PDGF?) may be important. It is noteworthy that there is reversal of normal blood flow originating in a central artery and extending to the periphery[18]. Although there is loss of typical lobular architecture, the overall structure of larger nodes somewhat resembles a normal liver lobule (pseudolobule): in and next to the fibrous septae, there are bile ducts and capillaries with non-fenestrated endothelia. The liver cell plates are one to two cells thick and may show slight fatty changes. However, the sinusoids have fenestrated endothelia and macrophages, as in normal liver tissue[19]. Because there is no convincing evidence of malignant transformation and the risk of bleeding is low (except in women taking oral contraceptives), resection is not mandatory[10,20].

### *Adenoma*

The epidemiology of adenomas shows a striking preponderance in women (74–93%), mainly after use of contraceptive pills. There are significant correlations between the cumulative dose of steroid hormones and the manifestation risk and size of adenomas. Whereas the incidence of adenomas has been estimated as being about 1–1.3 per million women in non-users of the ‘pill’, it is 3.4 per 100 000 in women taking oral contraceptives[21]. Adenoma may also develop after steroid intake. Pathogenetically, the occurrence of oestrogen- or steroid-receptors in adenoma cells has been demonstrated and may be the main pathogenetic event. Withdrawal of oestrogens or steroids may result in adenoma regression, but this can take many months. While oestrogen- and steroid-related adenomas are common, there are other aetiological factors, such as metabolic diseases (e.g. glycogenosis type I), familial conditions, cirrhosis and, finally, spontaneous types[10].

Macroscopically, hepatocellular adenomas show an average diameter of 6.3 cm with a range of 0.5–20 cm[22] but the mean diameter of resected specimens was usually more than 10 cm and the weight was more than 500 g[10]. Haemorrhage and necrosis or regressive pseudocysts may be dominant in some adenomas. Septa and peliosis may also occur occasionally.

Microscopically, adenomas consist of sheets of neohepatocytes in which four cell types can be distinguished[10]:

1. A type similar to normal liver cells;
2. Hydropic;
3. Pleomorphic; and
4. Glycogen-rich neohepatocytes.

Immunohistochemically, in adenomas, one can often find a partial or full substitution of fenestrated sinusoids by capillaries with ordinary non-fenestrated endothelial cells. This loss of fenestrated endothelia also entails a partial or subtotal loss of Kupffer cells; however, in some adenomas, the normal angioarchitecture and Kupffer cell density may be maintained. Thus, in a quantitative analysis of 7 adenomas, the content of Kupffer cells was lower than in the surrounding liver parenchyma in only 3 cases[23]. In minor biopsies, one therefore has to be cautious in using the loss of fenestrated endothelial cells and macrophages as a diagnostic clue in the histopathological differential diagnosis of liver tumours, and also in radiocolloid scintigraphy[24]. The often-reduced contrast in radiocolloid imaging may also result from the low perfusion of the lesion and the occurrence of central regression phenomena, such as necrosis and bleeding.

In a major metaanalysis, complications were found in more than one half of the adenoma patients; in about one third, they consisted of rupture and gross bleeding[25]. Nodule-within-nodule growth indicates malignancy. However, such a malignant transformation is very rare and is more often associated with adenomas resulting from an underlying metabolic disease. In view of the complications, adenomas should be resected if this can be done without causing mortality[26].

*Hepatocellular carcinoma (HCC)*

HCC is the most frequent carcinoma worldwide. The aetiological factors are:

1. Chronic hepatitis B infection in Japan and China (4.6–17/100 000);
2. Mycotoxins in Southern Africa and Mozambique (14.2–98.2/100 000), often in combination with viral hepatitis; and
3. Liver cirrhosis in Europe and USA (less than 3/100 000).

Alcoholic liver cirrhosis entails a fourfold increase in the risk of developing HCC. Among primary liver tumours, HCC dominates[10] with an incidence of 86.4%. Almost all HCC, except the fibrolamellar variant, express AFP; however, it is difficult to trace this marker in formalin-fixed, paraffin-embedded material.

Macroscopically, expansive, infiltrative and mixed types of HCC can be distinguished[27]. The expansive type usually develops within liver cirrhosis; it is encapsulated and infiltrates portal vessels very late in its course. This type includes uni- and multinodular subtypes, the latter probably representing primary multicentric as well as secondary intrahepatic metastasizing HCC. The infiltrating type accounts for one third of the cases and shows irregular borders; early portal vein invasion and intrahepatic metastases are typical of this subtype. There is a rare (5–12%) type of diffuse HCC[27] consisting of many nodules ranging from 0.5–1 cm.

'Small' or 'subclinical' HCC, which can be identified by US and AFP screening in patients at risk, is a tumour with fairly good prognosis (5 years' survival is about 50–80%). There are various definitions of small HCC: <2 cm (Japanese Association for Study of the Liver[28]); one HCC of 4.5 cm or a maximum of four HCC with a diameter of 3.5 cm[28]; or one HCC of 5 cm or two HCC with a total diameter of 5.5 cm[29].

Microscopically, HCC may show various aspects of cytopathological changes that are known to occur also in non-tumourous liver, e.g. extensive (focal) fatty changes. However, owing to the cellular heterogeneity within the same tumours, microscopic classifications are not very meaningful; this also applies with respect to the unfavourable prognosis (3–6 months survival) of advanced HCC. The only exception is fibrolamellar HCC which is characterized by manifestation at a young age, being of equal incidence in men and women and having a very protracted course. Under immunohistochemistry, the vascular channels in HCC are shown to be capillarized with a sparsely fenestrated endothelium and a significant reduction of Kupffer cells[30] (Figure 1.4). According to our own observations, the density of these capillary channels depends on the thickness of the neoplastic liver cell sheets and is very slight in solid growths.

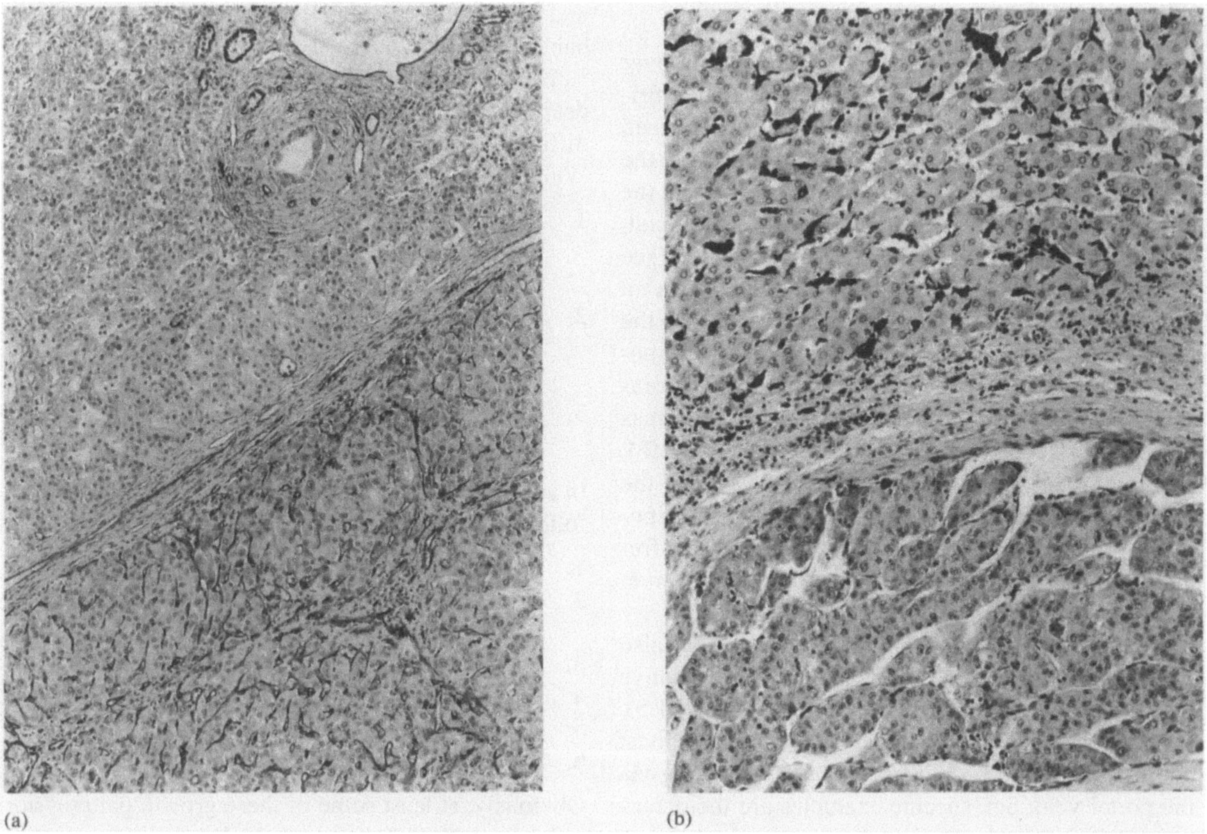


**Figure 1.4** Immunohistochemical distribution in HCC: (a) of non-fenestrated endothelia (CD 34) in the tumour (bottom) compared with normal liver (top) and (b) of macrophages (PGM1): loss in the tumour (bottom) and increase in the surrounding parenchyma (top). Avidin–Biotin, each 200×

## Histopathological differential diagnosis

The main differential diagnoses of hepatocellular lesions are FNH, liver cell adenoma and HCC. Some of the main features of the differential diagnosis between *FNH and adenoma* relate to the occurrence of a dysplastic artery, central scar, bile ducts and Kupffer cells in FNH, and the occurrence of bile ducts is of prime diagnostic importance here. The features of adenomas are the capsule, dysplasia, usually capillarization, necrosis, haemorrhage and rupture, as well as contraceptive use (see Table 1.2). The main distinctive features between *HCC and adenoma* are the presence of mitoses, cytological atypia, nodule-within-nodule, and an infiltrative margin or portal vein invasion in HCC, while degenerative changes and the occurrence of neohepatocytes are typical for adenoma[10]. Immunohistochemically, the Kupffer cell density[23] and the vascular pattern (own observations) may be focally normal in adenomas, whereas there is total capillarization and loss of Kupffer cells in HCC. The value of fine-needle biopsy in differential diagnosis will be discussed in another paper of this volume.

**Table 1.2 Morphological and clinical differences between FNH and liver adenoma**

| | *FNH* | *Adenoma* |
|---|---|---|
| Dysplastic artery | + | – |
| Central scar and septa | + | – |
| Bile duct proliferations | ++ | – |
| Kupffer cells | ++ | –/+ (!) |
| Capsule | (±) | ++ |
| Fatty changes | (±) | + |
| Dysplasia | – | + |
| Capillarization | – | (±) |
| Necrosis | – | (+) |
| Haemorrhage and rupture | – | (+) |
| Contraceptive pill | (+) | ++ |

*Metastases*

In a large series of 94 556 autopsies extending over 62 years, there were malignant extrahepatic primaries in 20.4%, of which 38% had metastasized into the liver[31]. Except for carcinomas of the prostate, the most frequent tumours produce the most frequent liver metastases, i.e. lung, colorectal, pancreatic, breast and stomach carcinomas (see Table 1.3). However, there are carcinomas with an unusually high incidence of liver metastases; the following tumours rank high among these: carcinomas of the gall bladder (77.6%), of the pancreas (70.4%), unknown primaries (57.0%), carcinomas of the colorectum (56.0%), of the breast (53.2%), and malignant melanoma (50.0%). In view of the biology of tumours, it is not surprising that carcinomas of the prostate and thyroid, although fairly frequent, do not produce a significant number of liver metastases.

Not only the type of the primary tumour, but also the age and sex of the patient influence the relative incidence of liver metastases[32,33] (see Figure 1.5). Except for metastases of frequent tumours, the most common metastases stem from tumours draining via the portal vein. Sex-specific examples are the occurrence of metastases from breast cancer in women, and from lung cancer in men because of smoking habits in males.

The macroscopic growth of liver metastases – despite large variations – shows typical patterns in different primary tumours. In the classification of Wuketich[34], three types were distinguished:

1. Large non-confluent metastases causing bulging of the hepatic capsule (e.g. metastases of colorectal carcinomas);
2. Medium-sized metastases of confluent type adapting to the liver capsule (e.g. metastases of breast carcinomas); and
3. Multiple (miliary) small metastases (e.g. small cell carcinomas and malignant melanoma).

In addition, Edmondson and Craig[31] distinguished the following subtypes:

1. Expanding, a. massive or b. uniform nodular,
2. Infiltrative, a. massive b. uniform multifocal or c. diffuse,
3. Surface spreading,
4. Incidental,
5. Miliary, and
6. Mixed or indeterminate.

Obviously, at least some of these growth patterns are influenced by different tumoural expression of cad-

**Table 1.3 Incidence of primary malignancies and liver metastases**

| *Site of primary* | *Primaries (n)* | *Liver metastases (n)* | *Relative incidence of metastases (%)* | *% of liver metastasis* |
|---|---|---|---|---|
| Lung | 682 | 285 | 41.8 | *24.8* (*1*) |
| Prostate | 333 | 42 | 12.6 | 3.6 (7) |
| Colon | 323 | 181 | *56.0* | *15.7* (2) |
| Breast | 218 | 116 | *53.2* | *10.1* (*4*) |
| Pancreas | 179 | 126 | *70.4* | *10.9* (*3*) |
| Stomach | 159 | 70 | 44.0 | *6.1* (*5*) |
| Kidney | 142 | 34 | 23.9 | 3.0 (9) |
| Cervix | 107 | 34 | 31.7 | 3.0 (10) |
| Unknown | 102 | 59 | *57.0* | *5.1* (*6*) |
| Ovary | 97 | 47 | 48.0 | 4.1 (7) |
| Thyroid | 70 | 12 | 17.1 | 1.0 (16) |
| Oesophagus | 66 | 20 | 30.3 | 1.7 (13) |
| Bladder and ureter | 66 | 25 | 37.9 | 2.2 (11) |
| Endometrium | 54 | 17 | 31.7 | 1.5 (15) |
| Melanoma | 50 | 25 | *50.0* | 2.2 (12) |
| Gall-bladder | 49 | 38 | *77.6* | 3.3 (8) |
| Testis | 45 | 20 | 44.4 | 1.7 (14) |
| Total | | 1151 | | |

Modified from Reference 31. Italic numbers represent tumours with an unusually high metastatic potential resulting in a high relative incidence of liver metastases.

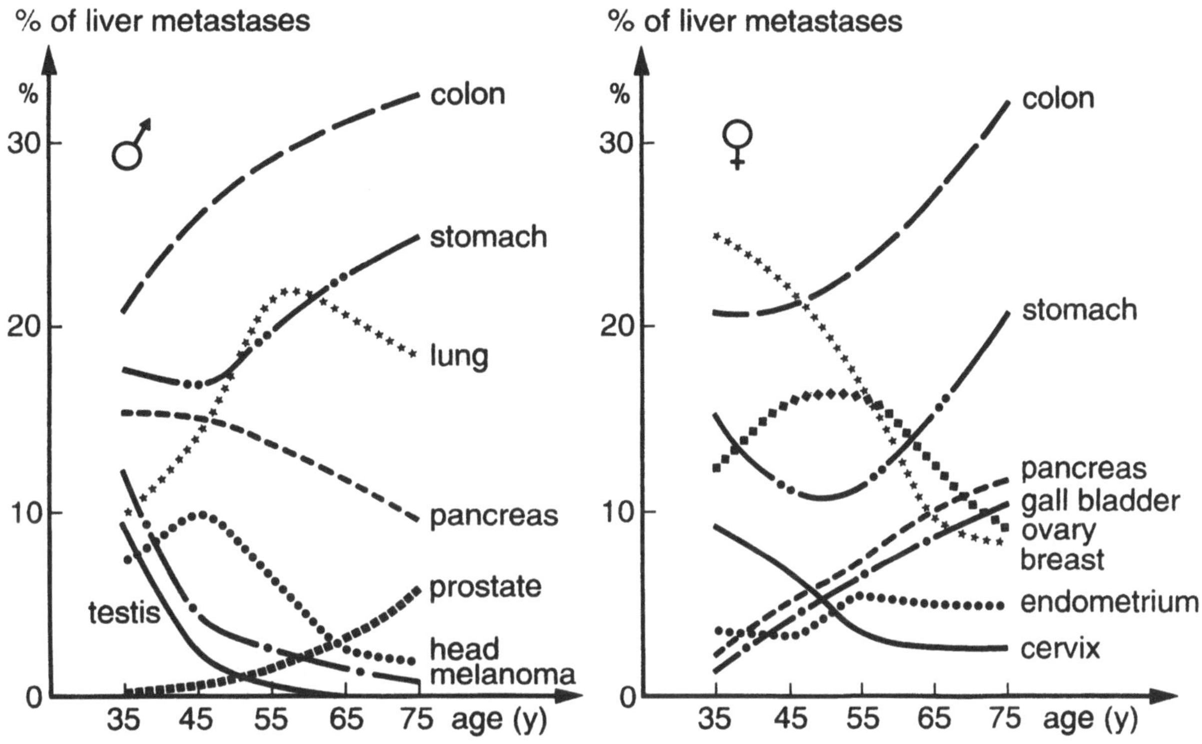


**Figure 1.5** Age- and sex-dependent incidence of liver metastases. Modified from References 32 and 33

herin molecules, fibrogenesis and probably also angiogenesis. Only a few morphometric data on the mean size of metastases in the various primaries have been obtained: in 57 autoptic livers with 11 581 metastases, the mean diameter was 1.0 cm[35]. However, in another selected series of 26 colorectal carcinomas with 1571 metastases, the mean diameter was 1.4 cm (range 0.2–9.0 cm)[36]. Since these cases might have been influenced by terminal tumour stages, a recent study[37] investigated only cases with a few liver metastases in order to determine the ratio of 'large' (>1 cm) to 'small' (<1 cm) metastases (Tables 1.4 and 1.5). In most tumours, the ratio between large and small metastases was 1:4, i.e. if one large metastasis is detected, one has to suspect that there are 4 more which may not be detected because of their small size. Only in colorectal carcinoma is this relationship of large:small metastases more favourable, being 1:1.6. This is probably the reason why the resection of metastases can be performed in colorectal carcinoma with a reasonable chance (20–30%) of long-term survival.

Immunohistochemical methods can be used for the analysis of histogenetic differentiation markers in order to distinguish the primary in an ever-growing proportion of metastases: for example, it is possible to trace malignant lymphomas (NHL: LCA, pan-B- and T-markers, light and heavy chains of immunoglobulins; Hodgkin's lymphoma: CD 30 and CD 15), thyroid primaries (thyroglobulin, calcitonin), carcinoma of the prostate (PSA and PSP), small cell carcinoma of the lung (NSE, Leu 7, CK 8, bombesin ±), carcinoid primary (NSE, Leu 7, CGA, CGC, synaptophysin, pancreatic hormones or gastrin), malignant melanoma (protein S100, HMB45), hepatocellular carcinoma (AFP ±; CK 18), cholangiocel-

**Table 1.4 Ratio of large (>1 cm) to small (<l cm) liver metastases with few metastatic nodules**

| *Total number of metastases (n)* | *Autopsy cases (n)* | *Ratio large:small metastases (n)* | *Relationship* |
|---|---|---|---|
| 1–3 | 10 | 14:45 | 1:3.2 |
| 4–9 | 19 | 72:285 | 1:3.9 |
| 10–24 | 3 | 60:239 | 1:3.9 |
| Total number | 32 | 132:524 | 1:3.9 |

From Reference 37

**Table 1.5 Ratio of large (>1 cm) to small (<1 cm) metastases in relation to the localization of the primary cancer**

| | *Total number of metastases (n)* | *Autopsy cases (n)* | *Ratio large:small metastases (n)* |
|---|---|---|---|
| Colorectum | 8 | 56 | 1:1.6 |
| Lung | 8 | 74 | 1:3.1 |
| All other sites | 26 | 615 | 1:4.5 |

From Reference 37

lular carcinoma (coexpression of CK 18 and 19), adenocarcinoma of ovary (Ca 125, no CK 20), adenocarcinoma of the colorectum (CK 20; no CK7; no Ca 125). As intestinal and gastric metaplasia play a distinctive role in carcinomas of the stomach, pancreas and gall bladder, it is not possible to distinguish them by their special profile of differentiation markers (e.g. expression of pepsinogens or mucins of gastric type). In some primaries, the histogenetic classification is more or less of academic interest, whereas, in other tumours, an effective therapy can now be offered.

### *References*


1. Wisse E, De Zanger RB, Charels K, Van der Smissen P, McKuskey RS. The liver sieve: Considerations concerning the structure and function of endothelial fenestrae, the sinusoidal wall and the space of Disse. Hepatology. 1985;5:683–92.
2. Bouwens L, Baekeland M, De Zanger R, Wisse E. Quantification, tissue distribution and proliferation kinetics of Kupffer cells in normal rat liver. Hepatology. 1986;6:718–22.
3. Sherlock S, Dooley J. Diseases of the liver and biliary system. 9th ed. London, Edinburgh, Boston, Melbourne, Paris, Berlin, Vienna: Blackwell Scientific Publications; 1993.
4. Horn T, Christoffersen P, Henriksen JH. Alcoholic liver injury: defenestration in non-cirrhotic livers. A scanning microscopic study. Hepatology. 1987;7:77–82.
5. Muro H, Shirasawa H, Kosugi I, Nakamura S. Defect of Fc receptors and phenotypical changes in sinusoidal endothelial cells in human liver cirrhosis. Am J Pathol. 1993; 143:105–20.
6. Wisse E. Ultrastructure and function of Kupffer cells and other sinusoidal cells in the liver. In: Wisse E, Knook DL, eds. Kupffer cells and other liver sinusoidal cells. Amsterdam: Elsevier/North-Holland Biomedical Press; 1977:33–60.
7. Fraser R, Day WA, Fernando NS. Review: The liver sinusoidal cells. Their role in disorders of the liver, lipoprotein metabolism and atherogenesis. Pathology. 1986;18:5–11.
8. Schmitt-Graeff A, Krueger S, Borchard F, Gabbiani G, Denk H. Modulation of a-smooth muscle actin and desmin expression in perisinusoidal cells of normal and diseased human liver. Am J Pathol. 1991;138:1233–42.
9. Lotz GW, Stahlschmidt M. Nicht-parasitäre parenchymatöse Lebercysten. Dtsch. Med. Wschr. 1987;112:1666–8.
10. Craig JR, Peters RL, Edmondson HA. Tumors of the liver and intrahepatic bile ducts. In: Atlas of tumor pathology. 2nd series, fascicle 26. Washington, DC: Armed Forces Institute of Pathology; 1988.
11. Melnick PJ. Polycystic liver, analysis of seventy cases. Arch Pathol. 1955;59:162–72.
12. Karhunen PJ. Benign hepatic tumours and tumour like conditions in men. J Clin Pathol. 1986;39:183–8.
13. Weiss H, Vorbeck S, Weiss A, Krahl C. Welche Bedeutung haben sonographisch entdeckte Lebertumoren? In: Hansmann M, Koischwitz D, Lutz H, Trier H-G, eds. Ultraschalldiagnostik '86. Berlin-Heidelberg-New-York-London-Paris-Tokyo: Springer; 1986:29–32.
14. Ishak KG, Rabin L. Benign tumors of the liver. Med Clin N Am. 1975;59:995–1013.
15. Kerlin P, Davis GL, McGill DB, Weiland LH, Adson MA, Sheedy PF. Hepatic adenoma and focal nodular hyperplasia: Clinical, pathologic, and radiologic features. Gastroenterology. 1983;84 (5 part 1):994–1002.
16. Schild H, Kreitner K-F, Thelen M, Groenninger J, Weber M, Stoerkel J, Eissner D. Fokal-nodulaere Hyperplasie der Leber bei 930 Patienten. Fortschr Roentgenstr. 1987; 147:612–8.
17. Wanless IR, Mawdsley C, Adams R. On the pathogenesis of focal nodular hyperplasia of the liver. Hepatology. 1985; 5:1194–200.
18. Schiff L, Schiff E, eds. Diseases of the liver. Philadelphia: Lippincott; 1983.
19. Zumdick M, Schmitt-Graeff A, Borchard F. Sinusoidale Wandzellen in Adenomen und fokalen nodulaeren Hyperplasien der Leber. Verh Dtsch Ges Path. 1991; 75:273.
20. Fechner RE, Roehm JOF. Angiographic and pathologic correlations of hepatic focal nodular hyperplasia. Am J Surg Pathol. 1977;1:217–24.
21. Rooks JB, Ory, HW, Ishak KG, Strauss LT, Greenspan JR, Hill AP, Tyler Jr CW. Epidemiology of hepatocellular adenoma. The role of oral contraceptive use. J Am Med Assoc. 1979;242:644–8.
22. Gold JH, Guzman IJ, Rosai J. Benign tumors of the liver. Pathologic examination of 45 cases. Am J Clin Pathol. 1978;70:6–17.
23. Goodman ZD, Mikel UV, Lubbers PR, Ros PR, Langloss JM, Ishak KG. Kupffer cells in hepatocellular adenomas. Am J Surg Pathol. 1987;11:191–6.
24. Salvo AF, Schiller A, Athanasoulis C, Galdabini J, McKusick KA. Hepatoadenoma and focal nodular hyperplasia: Pitfalls in radiocolloid imaging. Radiology. 1977; 125:451–5.
25. Kreitner KF, Thelen M, Schild H, Heintz S, Störkel S. Epidemiologie und klinische Aspekte der fokal-nodulären Hyperplasie der Leber. Dtsch Med Wschr. 1987; 112: 891–6.
26. Leese T, Farges O, Bismuth H. Liver cell adenomas. A 12 year surgical experience from a specialist hepato-biliary unit. Ann Surg. 1988;208:558–64.
27. Nakashima T, Kojiro M. Hepatocellular carcinoma. An atlas of its pathology. Tokyo–Berlin–Heidelberg–New York–London–Paris: Springer Verlag; 1987.
28. Okuda K, Ryu M, Tobe T. Surgical management of hepatoma. The Japanese experience. In: Wanebo HJ, ed. Hepatic and biliary cancer. New York–Basel: Marcel Dekker Inc; 1987:219–38.
29. Tang ZY, ed. Subclinical hepatocellular carcinoma. Berlin–Heidelberg–New York–Tokyo: Springer Verlag; 1985.
30. Haratake J, Scheuer PJ. An immunohistochemical and ultrastructural study of the sinusoids of hepatocellular carcinoma. Cancer. 1990;65:1985–93.
31. Edmondson HA, Craig JR. Neoplasms of the liver. In: Schiff L, Schiff ER, eds. Diseases of the liver. 6th ed. New York: JB Lippincott Company; 1987.

32. Bassermann R, Ludwig G, Hölzel D, Eder M. Haematogene Organmetastasen – welcher Primaertumor? Pathologe. 1984;5:13–20.
33. Borchard F. Pathologie der herdfoermigen Erkrankungen der Leber. Roentgenpraxis. 1989;42:266–70.
34. Wuketich S. Das Erscheinungsbild der Lebermetastasen und seine differentialdiagnostische Bedeutung (Morphologische Differentialdiagnose der Lebermetastasen). Beitr Path Anat. 1960;122:353–80.
35. Schulz W, Hort W. The distribution of metastases in the liver. Virchows Arch A (Pathol Anat). 1981;394:89–96.
36. Schulz W, Hagen Ch, Hort W. The distribution of liver metastases from colonic cancer. A quantitative post-mortem study. Virchows Arch A (Pathol Anat). 1985; 406: 279–84.
37. Schulz W, Borchard F. Groesse der Lebermetastasen bei geringer Metastasenzahl. Eine quantitative Studie an post-mortalen Lebern. Fortschr Roentgenstr. 1992;156:320–4.

# 2

# SONOGRAPHY OF FOCAL LIVER LESIONS

S. DELORME

## Introduction

Sonography is commonly the first imaging method used to assess the liver. A good knowledge of the diagnostic accuracy of the method is indispensable because other diagnostic procedures are applied according to the result of the ultrasound examination. Since sonography is applied very frequently, it reveals incidental findings which must subsequently be evaluated.

In a medicolegal autopsy study[1] (see Table 2.5), the prevalence of focal liver lesions was reported to be 51%, but lesions are detected in only 2–3% of sonographic examinations[2]. While the vast majority of lesions in the cited autopsy study was benign, malignant lesions account for 65–75% of lesions detected at sonography (see Table 2.6). This discrepancy is most probably due to:

— The preselection of patients (since sonography has become a routine procedure for cancer patients) and

— The size of the lesions. Most benign lesions in the cited autopsy study are too small to be detected, while malignant tumours eventually grow large enough.

A reliable diagnosis can often be made by sonomorphological criteria and information on the clinical background alone. Frequently, however, an additional imaging method or an invasive procedure is necessary to characterize a lesion and to decide upon the further clinical management of the patient.

This article gives a review of diagnostic criteria to characterize a lesion and points out pitfalls and limitations of the method as well as additional diagnostic procedures.

## Equipment and examination technique

3.5 MHz are standard for the examination of the entire organ. A 5-MHz transducer may be helpful to assess the superficial parts of the organ but only in very slim patients is it sufficient for an examination of the distal portions. Since the acoustic window is often very small (intercostal, subcostal), a sector scanner is preferred. A linear array may be used for the near field but only rarely reaches the entire subdiaphragmatic region. A curved array combines a wide distal field of view with a reasonable near field.

Common mistakes are:

— Neglect of the *remote parts* of the organ (left lateral segment, subdiaphragmatic parts and the inferior margin of the liver)

— Insufficient *image quality* due to insufficient acoustic window (cartilaginous ribs, linea alba, ligamentum falciforme or bowel gas may obscure the view).

— Neglect of the *near field* when a sector scanner is used.

A left lateral supine position is helpful, particularly in patients with a difficult subcostal access and for imaging of the porta hepatis.

## Malignant lesions

### *Primary liver tumours*

*Hepatocellular carcinoma* is rare among Caucasians and arises mainly in patients with liver cirrhosis or with chronic aggressive hepatitis. Small tumours

**Table 2.1 Ability of sonography to detect a liver tumour in the presence of cirrhosis (according to Dodd et al.)[8]. Preoperative detection of focal liver lesions in 100 cirrhotic patients scheduled for transplantation. Correlation with postoperative histopathology**

| *Histology* | *Sonography* | *Number of patients* | *Number of lesions* |
|---|---|---|---|
| Tumour | Tumour | 9 | 25 |
| Tumour | No tumour | 13 | 33† |
| | Total | 22 | 58* |
| No tumour | Tumour | 2 | |
| No tumour | No tumour | 76 | |
| | Total | 78 | |

* 46 hepatocellular carcinomas, 9 cholangiocarcinomas, 3 haemangiomas

(<3 cm) are commonly hypoechogenic and may show a slight distal echo enhancement. As the tumour grows, its echogeneity increases inhomogeneously[3] (Figure 2.1). Half of tumours of all sizes have a hypoechogenic rim ('halo')[4] and may be indistinguishable from metastases of an extrahepatic tumour. *Fibrolamellar carcinoma* is less commonly associated with pre-existing liver disease. This highly vascular tumour is echo-dense[5] and has a better prognosis.

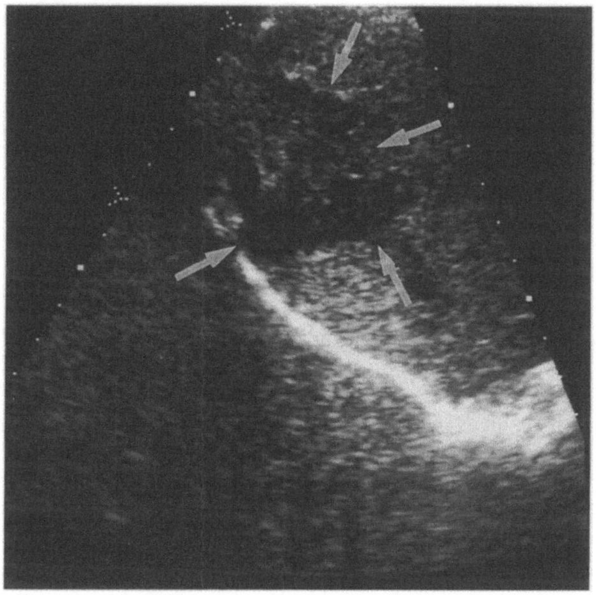

**Figure 2.1** Longitudinal subdiaphragmatic section, right liver lobe. Hepatocellular carcinoma due to Thorotrast exposure (arrows). Inhomogeneous echopattern, hypoechogenic rim, distal echo enhancement

*Cholangiocarcinoma* is not commonly associated with liver cirrhosis or chronic hepatitis. In our experience with Thorotrast patients, the tumour is mostly hypoechogenic and has a halo (Figure 2.2). Large tumours (5–20 cm) are hyper- or isoechogenic[6]. Obstructing tumours in the hepatic bifurcation (Klatskin tumours) are frequently missed by sonography if they grow in an infiltrative fashion. They mainly present with bilateral or unilateral dilatation of the intrahepatic bile ducts, where intraluminal parts of the tumour can be demonstrated at the site of obstruction[7].

The main *diagnostic problem* is that a tumour is difficult to detect in a liver which often has a grossly inhomogeneous echostructure due to the pre-existing cirrhosis. Additional fatty infiltration causes strong attenuation and makes it particularly difficult to assess the far field. If the liver is shrunken due to the cirrhosis, only a small acoustic window may remain because of bowel interposition. As a consequence, sonography performs badly with a detection rate of less than 50% of liver tumours in presence of cirrhosis[8].

The *differential diagnosis* of a suspected lesion is often difficult. Not infrequently, a lesion initially thought to be a metastasis turns out to be a primary liver tumour at biopsy[9]. In cirrhosis, the alteration of the liver structure by regenerative changes may even

**Table 2.2 Differential diagnosis of the primary liver tumour**

| *Sono-morphology* | *Differential diagnosis* | *Signs in common* | *Decision criteria* | *Additional studies* |
|---|---|---|---|---|
| Small, echo-poor | Cyst | Distal echo enhancement | Distal wall enhancement | CT with iv contrast |
| Large, echo-rich | Haemangioma | | Halo in malignant lesions | Dynamic CT, blood pool scan, MRI |
| Complex echo structure | FNH, adenoma | | Cirrhosis?<br><br>Age, sex, contraceptives? | Dynamic CT, HIDA scan |
| Any sono-morphology | Metastasis | Halo | Extrahepatic primary tumour? Metastases rare in cirrhosis | FNB |

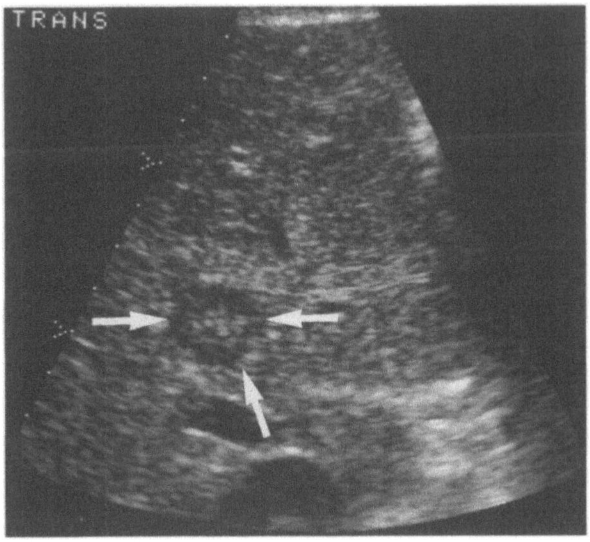


**Figure 2.2** Epigastric transverse section. Isoechogenic cholagiocarcinoma with hypoechogenic halo (arrows)

mimic a tumour[8]. Table 2.2 gives an overview of differential diagnostic criteria. Besides information about an extrahepatic primary tumour, it is important to know whether the patient has liver cirrhosis, because metastases in cirrhotic livers are rare[10]. Ultimately, most suspicious lesions must be confirmed by fine-needle biopsy.

*Sonographic screening for risk groups*

Despite its limitations, sonography is applied in screening of patients at risk for liver cancer because it is non-invasive and cost-effective. In short-term cohort screening studies using ultrasound on patients with liver cirrhosis, the annual incidence of primary liver tumours is reported to be 2–10%[11–13]. In a 10-year study on Thorotrast patients at the German Cancer Research Center[14], the average annual incidence of liver neoplasms was 1.5% which is still a considerable risk. Therefore, regular sonographic studies for patients at risk for primary liver tumours because of cirrhosis is recommended and appears to be superior to screening with $\alpha$-fetoprotein (AFP) alone[11]. Four screening studies are summarized in Table 2.7. In our experience, ultrasonography and CT are a useful combination in addition to biochemical tests. MRI should be applied if both methods fail to exclude the possibility of a tumour.

*Metastases*

Metastases can present with virtually every sonomorphological appearance. The echopatterns are classified as follows:

— *Hypoechogenic, hyperechogenic* (Figure 2.3) or *isoechogenic* to the surrounding liver tissue.

— *Hypoechogenic halo* in lesions of any echogeneity. Isoechogenic lesions are only visible because of the halo (Figure 2.4) or if they distort the liver surface, displace or invade vessels, etc.

— *Central echolucent zone* (Figure 2.5) due to necrosis (in large metastases) or in true cystic lesions (rare, e.g. in metastases due to ovary cancer).

— *Solitary* or *multiple* lesions. In cases with a *diffuse distribution*, single lesions are almost invisible: a grossly inhomogeneous echo-structure of the liver is the only clue to the diagnosis.

The echo structure rarely helps to identify the primary tumour. Since many hyperechogenic metastases are due to a gastrointestinal or breast tumours[15], the initial workup of the patient may focus on these organs. The value of further consideration is doubtful since, in 20% of patients with multiple hepatic metastases, different echo-patterns have been observed simultaneously[16].

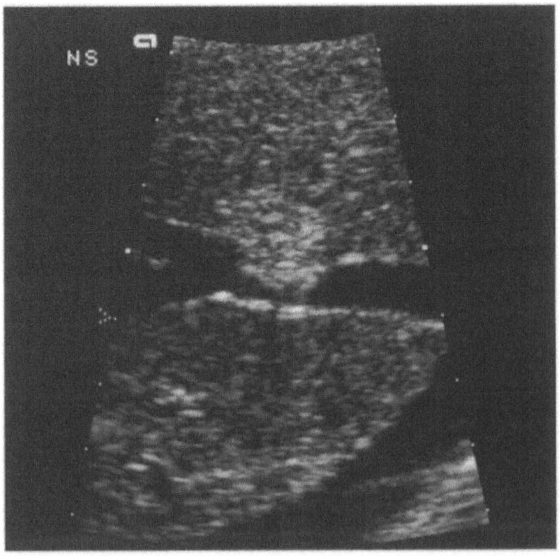


**Figure 2.3** Transverse section, left liver lobe. Hyperechogenic metastasis due to renal carcinoma which invades a hepatic vein

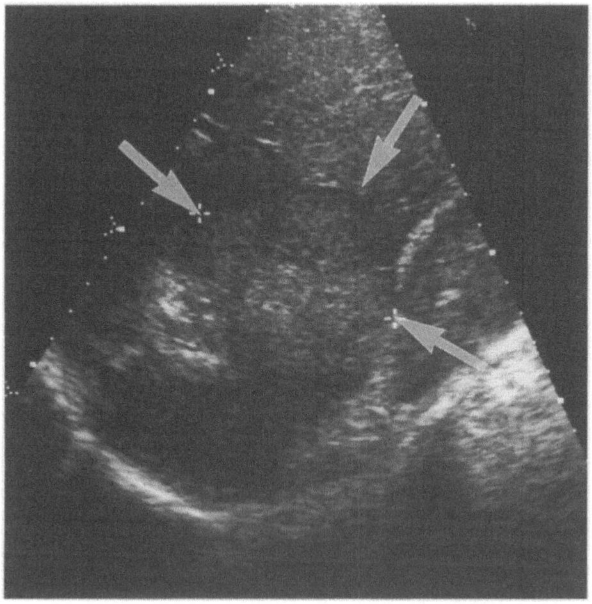

**Figure 2.4** Longitudinal section, mid-clavicular line. Isoechogenic metastasis (arrows) with a thin halo which is just visible

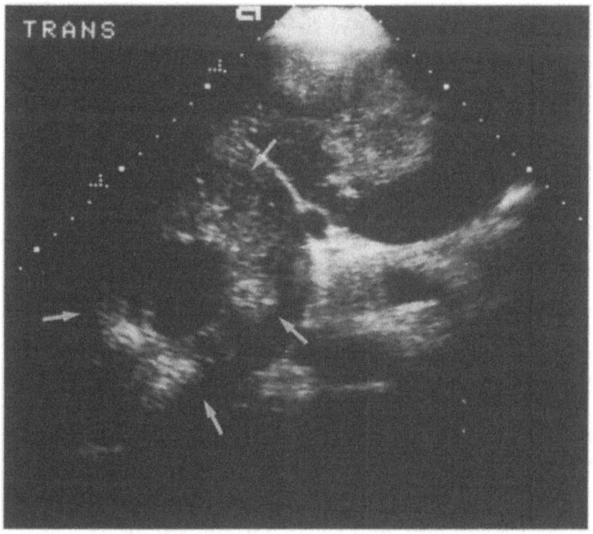


**Figure 2.5** Epigastric transverse section. Hyperechogenic metastases due to bronchus carcinoma (arrows). Central necrosis

The echo-pattern of metastases has been correlated to histomorphological features:

— *Vascularity*. Autopsy studies have demonstrated a high degree of vascularity in hyperechogenic lesions while hypovascular metastases were more commonly echo-poor[17].

— *Fibroplastic reaction, calcifications* and *fatty infiltration* increase the echogeneity. These processes are observed during growth of a lesion as well as during chemotherapy (Figure 2.6)[18].

— *Necrosis* may cause echolucent areas inside a lesion.

— Metastases preserving a *glandular pattern* of the organ of origin (such as gastrointestinal tumours) may appear echo-rich.

The *halo* may be just visible as a thin line or present as a broad hypoechogenic rim. Its histomorphological correlate is controversial. According to Marchal et al[19], the halo corresponds not to the lesion itself but to the surrounding liver tissue which is compressed by the tumour. Wernecke et al.[20] reported that the halo represents the rapidly proliferating tumour periphery which has not yet undergone regressive changes.

## Differential diagnosis of liver metastases

A metastasis may be mimicked by a variety of benign lesions. Table 2.3 gives an overview of the differential diagnosis of metastases versus benign changes. Again, it is important to know whether the patient has a liver

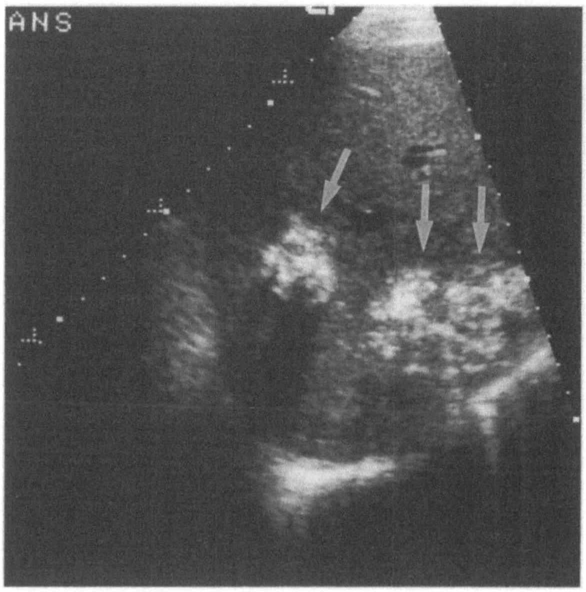


**Figure 2.6** Transverse subcostal section. Patient with colon carcinoma metastatic to the liver treated with chemotherapy. Multiple calcified metastases (arrows)

**Table 2.3 Differential diagnosis of metastases versus benign focal liver lesions**

| *Sonomorphology of the metastasis* | *Differential diagnosis* | *Signs in common* | *Decision criteria* | *Additional studies* |
|---|---|---|---|---|
| Echo-rich | Haemangioma | Smooth border | Halo in metastasis<br><br>Geographic border in haemangioma | Dynamic CT, blood pool scan, angiography |
| | Lipoma | | | CT |
| | Local fatty infiltration | | Geographic border, no expansion or destruction in fatty infiltration | Colloid scan |
| Echo-poor | Cyst | Internal echoes in cyst (scanner setting?) | Typical signs of a cyst | CT with i.v. contrast |
| | FNH | | | CT with i.v. contrast, HIDA scan |
| | Focal non-steatosis | | Geographic border, no expansion or destruction in focal non-steatosis | CT, colloid scan |
| Central echolucent zone | Abscess | | Clinical picture | FNB, drainage white blood cell scan |
| Halo | Adenoma (rare!) | | | FNB (beware of haemorrhage!), colloid and HIDA scan |

cirrhosis or an extrahepatic malignancy. A lateral shadow sign, a distal amplification without a distal wall enhancement and the presence of regions with different echogeneity within one lesion (mosaic pattern) favour liver cancer. A small hyperechogenic lesion is likely to be a metastasis rather than a primary liver tumour[21]. If there are multiple lesions, the diagnosis is probably metastastatic disease rather than primary liver tumour, but multicentric liver cancer does occur.

A halo in a benign lesion is rare and is strongly indicative of malignancy[22–24], but it occurs in both primary and secondary liver tumours. Similarly, a central echolucent zone within a solid lesion is most commonly a central necrosis and indicates malignancy. An abscess must be considered for differential diagnosis but has only a thin wall.

A smoothly marginated liquid lesion without a wall is a reliable sign of a cyst and excludes malignancy. Hypoechogenic lesions in an otherwise normoechogenic liver merit a definite workup because benign lesions are only rarely echo-poor (adenoma, focal nodal hyperplasia)[25].

## Value of sonography for the detection of metastases

The ability of sonography to detect metastatic disease is limited by the size of the lesions. In an autopsy study, 154 metastases with an average diameter of

**Table 2.4 Sensitivity of sonography, CT and MRI to detect metastases (according to Wernecke et al.[27])**

| *Lesion size* | *Sonography* | *CT* | *MRI* |
|---|---|---|---|
| All lesions | 53% | 68% | 63% |
| <1 cm | 20% | 49% | 31% |

CT unenhanced, after rapid injection of i.v. contrast medium as well as delayed scans, MRI in T1 and T2 weighted spin-echo sequences. 75 patients with gastrointestinal tumours. Gold standard: intraoperative finding including intraoperative sonography

1 cm were found in 75 livers[26]. In 47 livers (62%), the mean diameter was 0.4–2 cm. Therefore, ultrasound must be expected to miss a considerable subset of lesions. In addition, metastases are easily missed due to:

— The patient's constitution (obesity, fatty liver, diaphragmatic relaxation, bowel interposition);

— Insufficient examination technique;

— Insufficient contrast between the lesions and the liver; and

— Metastases in problematic regions: subdiaphragmatically, adjacent to the falciform ligament, in the caudate lobe, at the left lateral border or superficially, close to the transducer.

In clinical studies, the performance of ultrasound is disappointing. Sonography detects only 53% of all lesions and 20% of metastases smaller than 1 cm. CT with i.v. contrast agent infusion appears to be superior but requires a meticulous examination technique[27]. One must conclude that the value of sonography for the *exclusion* of metastases is only limited, mainly because of its inability to detect small lesions. However, the clinical value of sonography is to positively *demonstrate* liver involvement in cancer and thereby to influence clinical management.

**Table 2.5 Frequency of focal liver lesions at mediolegal autopsy (according to Karhunen[1]) of 95 men without history of related disease**

| *Finding* | *Frequency (%)* | *Size (cm)* |
|---|---|---|
| Haemangioma | 20 | 0.5–2 |
| Adenoma | 1 | 0.6 |
| FNH | 3 | 0.8–6.5 |
| Metastasis (colon cancer) | 1 | 0.5–2 |
| Benign biliary tumours (adenomas, microhamartomas) | 27 | 0.03–0.5 |
| Others | 2 | |
| Total (2 patients had lesions with multiple histologies) | 51 | |

**Table 2.6 Frequency of focal liver lesions at sonography in hospitalized patients (according to Weiss[2])**

| | *Frequency (%) 1987* $n = 75\,840$ | *Frequency (%) 1990* $n = 6208$ |
|---|---|---|
| Metastases | 1.58 | 1.97 |
| Haemangiomas | 0.03 | 0.79 |
| Fatty changes | 0.003 | 0.24 |
| FNH | 0.0013 | 0.06 |
| Calcifications | | 0.08 |
| Adenomas | 0.0065 | 0.016 |
| Primary liver tumours | 0.011 | |
| Cysts | 0.52 | 0.05 |
| Other benign findings | | 0.11 |
| Total benign solid | 0.41 | 1.35 |
| Total | 2.15 | 3.32 |

Ultrasound plays no role in the detection of liver or spleen involvement in *malignant lymphoma*, since the infiltration pattern is diffuse in 90%. In only 10% is the involvement focal and permits detection by sonography. Involved regions are mostly echo-poor, occasionally confluent and have no halo sign[28].

## Benign liver lesions

### *Focal nodal hyperplasia (FNH) and liver adenoma*

Most reports on imaging of *FNH* suffer from small series because this is a rare lesion. If not otherwise stated, the following figures refer to a meta analysis on 930 patients by Schild et al.[29]. The sonomorphology of FNH is extremely variable. The size may range from few millimeters to 20 cm. The 'central scar' carrying supplying vessels is occasionally visible as a convergence of bright septae-like structures (Figure 2.7). An FNH may distort the liver surface (Figure 2.8) and even present as a pedunculated tumour. Often it is an incidental finding at sonography for other indications. 94% of FNH are detected by sonography but second or third lesions are missed in 13%.

The hallmark of FNH is a positive *HIDA scan* (in 91%) and a strong and early enhancement during *dynamic CT* (in 94% within the first 2 minutes)[29,30]. These features are sufficient to exclude a malignant tumour[31]. Unfortunately, these properties are frequently shared by *liver adenoma* which carries the risk of malignant transformation and intra-abdominal bleeding. Different features of FNH and adenoma are reported with CT showing a central scar in 66% of FNH. The role of *colloid scintigraphy* which shows an uptake in 63% of FNH is controversial. An at-least residual uptake is reported in up to 23%[32]. One may assume an FNH with some confidence in presence of a pedunculated tumour, a central scar on CT and a positive colloid uptake or central vessels with high flow velocities shown by *Doppler sonography*. In *gradient-echo MRI*, these vessels may appear as centrally located hyperintense spots (Ros PR, personal communication). *Fine-needle biopsy* (FNB) may be helpful but must be managed with care since subcapsular adenomas tend to bleed into the peritoneal cavity and even necessitate surgical intervention.

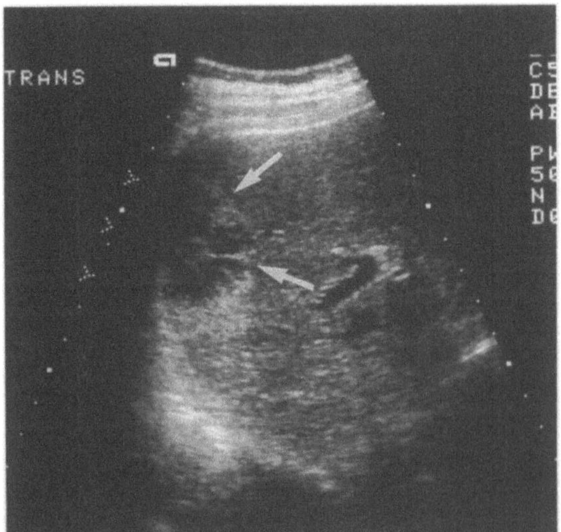


**Figure 2.7** Subcostal transverse section. Hyperechogenic FNH with an echo-dense rim (arrows)

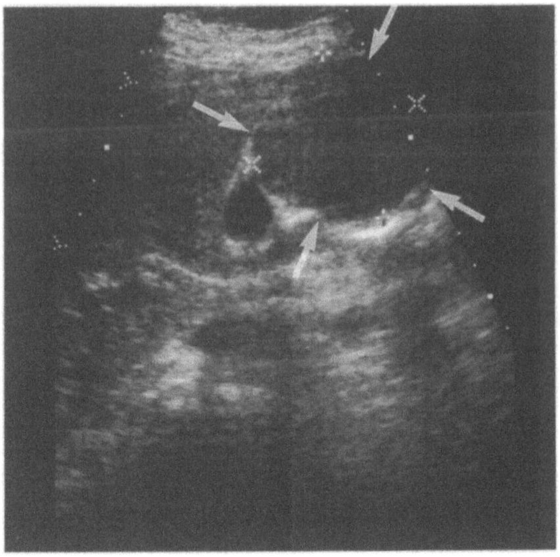

**Figure 2.8** Epigastric transverse section. Focal nodal hyperplasia in the 4th segment (arrows). Isoechogenic tumour causing a bulge in the liver surface and compressing the gall-bladder

### *Haemangioma*

Haemangiomas are found in 7% of careful autopsies[1]. Their size may range from few millimeters to several centimeters. They are a common incidental finding during liver sonography of any indication. Diagnostic problems arise mainly in cancer patients referred for staging. Criteria of 'typical' and 'atypical' haemangiomas are listed in Table 2.8. However,

**Table 2.7 Ultrasound screening of patients at increased risk for liver cancer**

| *Risk factor* | *Patients* | *Sonographies* | *Interval* | *Tumours detected* | *Reference* |
|---|---|---|---|---|---|
| Cirrhosis | 157 | | 2 years | 15 | Cottone et al.[11] |
| Cirrhosis | 214 | 214 | 1 year | 20 | Tremolda et al.[13] |
| Cirrhosis | 660 | 2004 | 19 months | 22 | Tanaka et al.[12] |
| Thorotrast | 334 | 741 | 10 years | 53 | Bast.[14] |

**Table 2.8 Criteria of typical and atypical haemangiomas according to Rettenmaier[51]. Frequency of findings according to Nelson and Chezmar[52]**

| *Typical* | *Atypical* |
|---|---|
| Hyperchogenic (67–70%) | Size >4 cm |
| Homogeneous (58–73%) | Inhomogeneous with hypoechogenic or echolucent components |
| Round, oval or geographical shape | Polycyclic contour |
| No halo | Halo (extremely uncommon) |
| Distal reverberations (up to 77%) | Space occupying features |
| Hyperechogenic margins | |
| Sharp margins (77–92%) | |
| Multiple lesions | |
| Site adjacent to vessels | |

even a 'typical' haemangioma (e.g. a small round lesion) may be indistinguishable from a metastasis. Occasionally, secondary signs of malignancy, like vessel invasion, enable a correct diagnosis (Figure 2.3). The most reliable sign is a 'geographic' border and a peripheral echo enhancement (Figure 2.9). A halo virtually excludes a haemangioma but may be imitated by an adjacent vessel. In *giant haemangiomas* (>4 cm), unsharp margins and a mixed echo pattern with hypoechogenic and hyperechogenic regions are common, requiring differentiation from FNH, adenoma and malignant liver tumours. When examining a haemangioma, the examiner must resist the inclination to misinterpret or even neglect other intrahepatic lesions because a haemangioma may very well be present together with a malignant liver lesion at another site.

In lesions of more than 1.5 cm, a definite diagnosis may be achieved with *dynamic CT*[33]. Since the latter carries a high local radiation dose and its results for smaller lesions are often unsatisfactory, we prefer to perform *blood pool scintigraphy* with SPECT, which is almost specific[34,35]. *MRI* is used with increasing frequency. So far, quantitative studies have failed to demonstrate a T2 threshold with sufficient sensitivity and specificity for differentiation from metastasis[36]. In clinical practice, however, a persistently high (isointense to liquor) or even increasing T2 intensity with longer echo times has proved a reliable criterion.

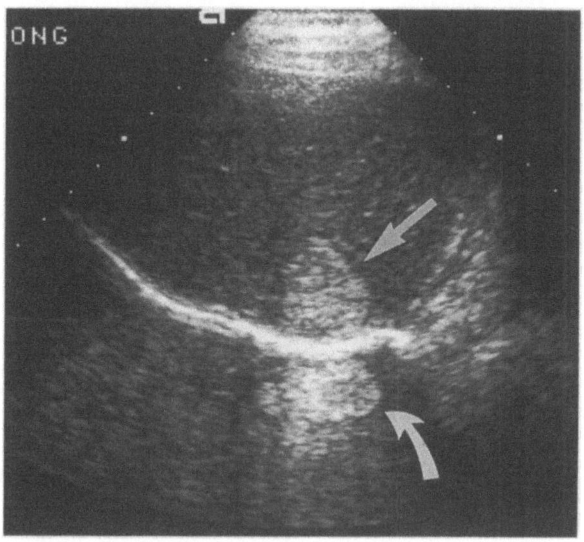


**Figure 2.9** Transverse subcostal section. Subdiaphragmatic haemangioma (straight arrow) with mirror artifact (curved arrow)

The most invasive approach is *hepatic angiography* which should be restricted to selected cases only. Under no circumstances should a potentially curable therapy be withheld because of an unclarified liver lesion.

### *Lipoma and angiomyolipoma*

These benign tumours are rare and appear as sharply delineated and echo-rich lesions. They can be reliably diagnosed with CT, showing negative density values (HU)[37,38].

### *Cysts*

Cysts are common incidental findings during sonography. They are frequently associated with renal or pancreatic cysts. Typically, they are echolucent with a distal wall enhancement, a distal echo enhancement and a lateral shadow sign and they lack a depictable solid wall. Small septae may be visible inside the cyst. With state-of-the-art scanners, cysts only seldom cause diagnostic problems. However,

- In a normal (relatively echo-poor) liver, a cyst may escape detection because of *insufficient contrast*.
- With *small cysts*, a distal wall enhancement and a lateral shadow sign are difficult to demonstrate.
- Under technically difficult conditions, internal echoes are difficult to eliminate, particularly in the *near field*. Care must be taken to optimize the scanner settings because even an inappropriate focus may obscure the cyst signs (Figure 2.10).
- A weak distal echo enhancement may also be encountered in malignant liver tumours or, more seldom, in metastases.

*CT* is often sufficient for clarification and shows a sharply delineated lesion of 0–20 HU without contrast enhancement or a solid wall. Small cysts require thin slices (>5 mm) because of partial volume effect. Conversely, sonography is often a helpful adjunct to clarify doubtful lesions on hepatic CT[39].

### *Echinococcus*

Any cystic lesion with internal reproducible echoes, solid components or wall calcifications must be suspected to be due to *Echinococcus cysticus (granulosus)*. The typical appearance of a 'cyst inside a cyst' is not always present. *Echinococcus alveolaris* presents as a poorly delineated and inhomogeneous tumour, sometimes with calcifications, mimicking a malignant liver tumour. Calcifications may dominate the image and obscure the underlying solid lesions. A diagnostic puncture carries the severe risk of intra-abdominal spread and anaphylactic reactions in a

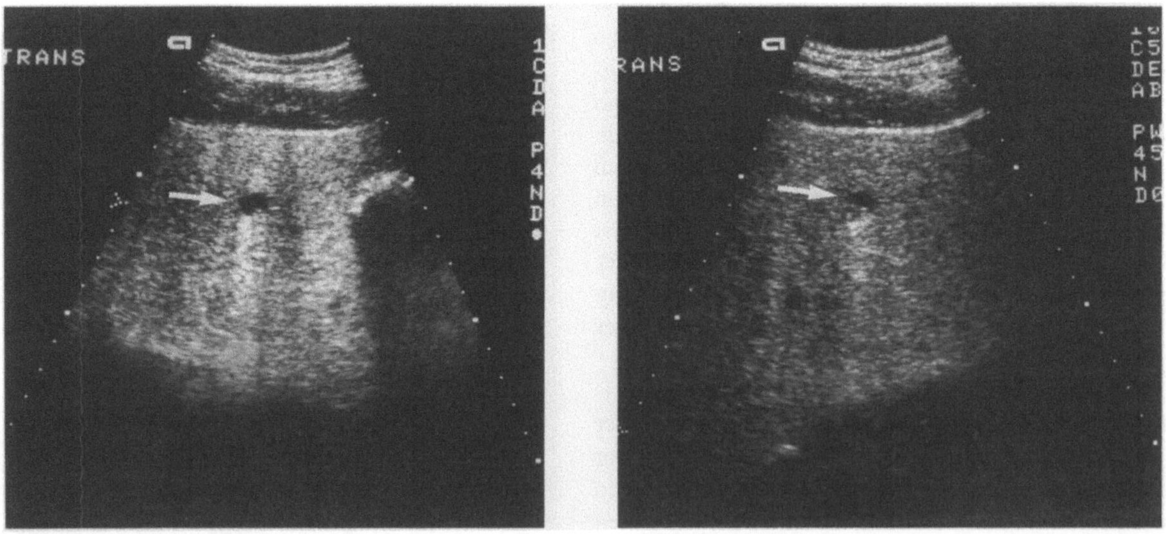

**Figure 2.10** Longitudinal section, mid-clavicular line. Liver cyst (arrow) in a patient with diffuse hepatic fatty infiltration. With correct setting, an echolucent lesion with distal echo enhancement and a lateral shadow sign can be demonstrated (left). With identical setting but incorrect focusing, the typical sonomorphology is obscured. The cyst now resembles a solid lesion (right)

case of cyst rupture. Therefore, open surgery is often preferred if imaging and lab tests are suggestive of echinococcosis.

### *Abscess*

Any cystic lesion with a solid wall is suspected of being either a necrotic metastasis or an abscess. A fresh abscess typically shows internal echoes, but old lesions may be completely echolucent. The internal border is often irregular in both and lacks a distal wall enhancement, though a distal echo enhancement is commonly visible and more pronounced than in any solid lesion (Figure 2.11). This criterion is important in cases when the abscess membrane is too thin to be detectable. Often, the diagnosis is straightforward because of the *clinical picture* (malaise, fever, leucocytosis, upper abdominal tenderness). Further procedures include *CT, a white blood cell scan* and a *pucture and drainage* under sonographic guidance, which is also a therapeutic measure.

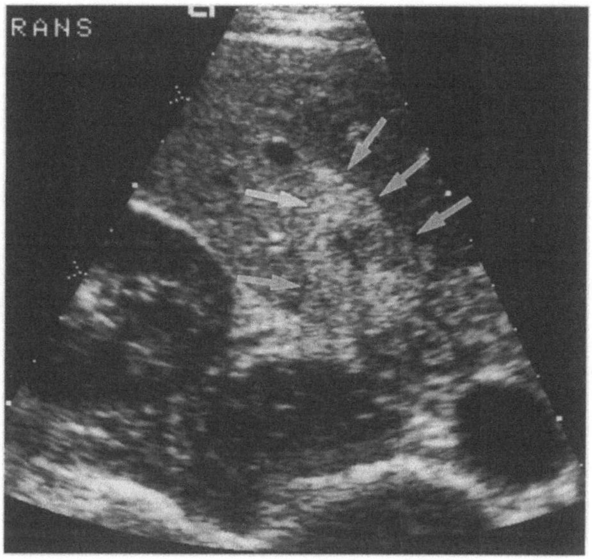


**Figure 2.12** Transverse subcostal section. Hyperechogenic liver due to fatty infiltration. Focal increase of fat (arrows) with geographic border. Note that the left side of this liver lobe (right side of the image) appears darker due to inhomogeneous fat distribution

### *Pseudotumours*

Focal fatty infiltration is rather uncommon and appears as an echo-rich region with a sharp border (Figure 2.12). These zones may expand and coalesce[40] but do not displace or even destroy anatomical structures. By analogy, areas spared from an otherwise generalized fatty infiltration (focal non-steatosis) appear hypeoechogenic in a hyperechogenic liver. Typically, these pseudotumours have a sharp and geographic (sometimes triangular) border and are located in the 4th segment close to the gall-bladder (41%) (Figure 2.13), the portal vein (37%) or superficially[41]. Only in 50% is a focal non-steatosis reproducible in *CT*, potentially because echo-density is not only a function of quantitative fat content but also of fat distribution[42,43]. Higher detection rates may result with fourth-generation scanners. In cases of large pseudotumours, *colloid scintigraphy* shows no decreased uptake and is the most appropriate way to exclude malignancy.

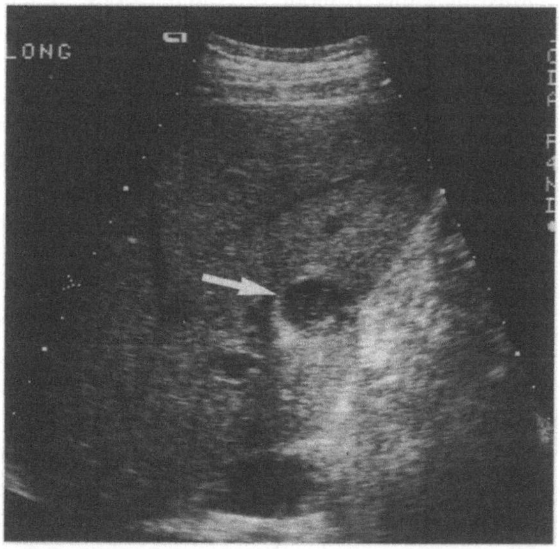


**Figure 2.11** Longitudinal section, anterior axillary line. Liver abscess in a patient with ascending cholangitis (arrow). Note the presence of internal echoes and a marked distal echo enhancement

## Extended applications

### *Intraoperative sonography*

Because of its unimpaired access without attenuation by the abdominal wall and the use of higher transducer frequencies, intraoperative sonography is superior for the detection of small metastases[44–47] and serves as a gold standard to assess the capabilities of other imaging modalities[27]. Since up to 40% of sono-

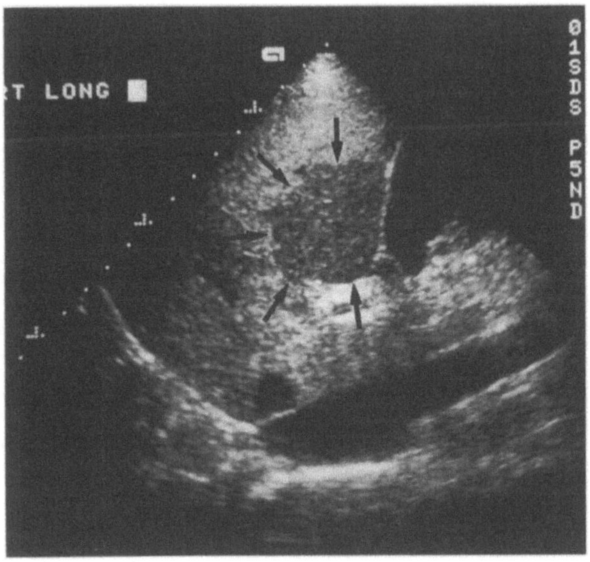


**Figure 2.13** Longitudinal section, mid-clavicular line. Focal non-steatosis (arrows) in typical localization.

graphically detected lesions are neither visible nor palpable to the surgeon[45], intraoperative sonography has become a standard diagnostic procedure for oncological abdominal surgery.

*Doppler sonography*

Since even slow blood flow in tumours can be made visible with highly sensitive colour Doppler scanners, the role of this imaging modality for differential diagnosis is being increasingly investigated. In liver imaging, however, Doppler sonography is hampered by serious methodological problems:

— Frequencies as low as 3.5 MHz are needed to penetrate into deeper regions of the organ. This *decreases the sensitivity to slow flow*. Even with 3.5 MHz, weak signal from low volume flow are hardly detectable because of considerable ultrasound attenuation.

— Transmitted cardiac pulsations cause disturbing *flashing artifacts* when a slow flow setting is used, particularly in the left lobe.

Since branches of the portal and hepatic veins are commonly visible with colour Doppler, vessels displacement or invasion by a tumour can be demonstrated. Metastases and haemangiomas normally show no detectable intratumoural flow because of slow velocities and small flow volume. Primary liver tumours and FNH frequently show considerable vascularization[48,49]. Unfortunately, this imaging modality does not help to solve common diagnostic problems like the differential diagnosis between haemangioma and metastasis.

*Ultrasound-guided fine-needle biopsy (FNB)*

The diagnostic accuracy of ultrasound-guided FNB depends on the depth and the size of the lesion. Since a lesion of less than 2 cm size is difficult to hit, even under sonographic guidance, a negative biopsy result must be critically weighted. According to Buscarini et al.[50], the sensitivity of this procedure is 92–95% and the negative predictive value is 83%, warranting a repeat biopsy if malignancy is still suspected despite a negative cytological result. Combination of cytology and histology increases the sensitivity to 97% (metastasis or liver cancer) to 100% (lymphoma), provided needle localization is accurate.

*Enhancing lesion detection*

Despite a high standard of equipment and staff, the value of ultrasonography for liver screening in patients with cancer or cirrhosis is severely limited by its inability to depict small lesions. Intravascular ultrasound contrast media are undergoing clinical trials which are expected to increase the lesion/liver contrast on either B-mode or colour Doppler images due to differences in vascularity. According to our own observations in patients with primary or secondary malignant liver tumours, there is a marked signal increase in the tumour periphery with colour Doppler after injection of contrast medium. Though this enhancement may help to depict single lesions, the method is still limited by the rapid decay of the vascular enhancement which prohibits a long and thorough examination.

Half of the population carries a benign liver lesion[1]. The series reported by Weiss[2] shows that, between 1987 and 1990, the detection rate of benign and malignant lesions has improved from 2.15% to 3.32%, most probably due to better equipment. However, an increased detection of benign lesions accounts for more than half the improvement. In the 1990 series reported by Weiss, the workup required was: 53 procedures (CT, FNB, laparoscopy, surgery and angiography) for 122 patients with metastases and 25 procedures (CT, laparoscopy, scintigraphy) for

83 patients with benign conditions. Any non-specific improvement of the diagnostic sensitivity of ultrasound as with contrast media (and without additional information to characterize a lesion) will potentially lead to an increased detection of benign liver lesions and thereby initiate further workup. More specific contrast media are under development but not ready for application (Balzer Th., personal communication).

## *References*


1 Karhunen PJ. Benign hepatic tumours and tumour like conditions in men. J Clin Pathol. 1986;39:183.
2. Weiss H. Sonographische Artdiagnostik tumoröser Leberveränderungen. Ultraschall Klin Prax. 1993;6:257.
3. Yoshikawa J, Matsui O, Takashima T, Ida M, Takanaka T, Kawamura I, Kakuda K, Miyata S. Fatty metamorphosis in hepatocellular carcinoma: radiologic features in 10 cases. Am J Roentgenol. 1988;15:717.
4. Choi BI, Kim CW, Han MC, Kim CY, Lee SS, Kim ST, Kim YI. Sonographic characteristics of small hepatocellular carcinoma. Gastrointest Radiol. 1989;14:255
5. Bedi DG, Kumar R. Morettin LB, Gourlex K. Fibrolamellar carcinoma of the liver: CT, ultrasound and angiography. Eur J Radiol. 1988;8:109.
6. Ros PR, Buck JL, Goodman ZD, Ros AMV, Olmsted WW. Intrahepatic cholangiocarcinoma: radiologic–pathologic correlation. Radiology. 1988;167:689.
7. Choi BI, Lee JH, Han MC, Kim SH, Yi JG, Kim CW. Hilar cholangiocarcinoma: comparative study with sonography and CT. Radiology. 1989;172:689.
8. Dodd GDI, Miller WJ, Baroin RL, Confer SR. Sonographic screening of cirrhotic livers: a prospective study. Radiology. 1990;181:153.
9. Reuß J, Seitz K. Sonographische Diagnostik des hepatozellulären Karzinoms. Ultraschall. 1989;10:111.
10. Seitz G. Warum sind Metastasen in zirrhotischen Lebern so selten? Ultraschall. 1989;10:123.
11. Cottone M, Turri M, Caltogirone M, Maringhini A, Scarrino E, Virdone R, Gusco R, Orlando A, Marino L, Pagliaro L. Early detection of hepatocellular carcinoma associated with cirhosis by ultrasound and alfafetoprotein: a prospective study. Hepatogastroenterology. 1988;35:101.
12. Tanaka S, Kitamura T, Nakanishi K, Okuda S, Yamazaki H, Hiyama T, Fujiimoto I. Effectiveness of periodic checkup by ultrasonography for the early diagnosis of hepatocellular carcinoma. Cancer. 1990;66:2210.
13. Tremolda F, Benevegnùi L, Drago C, Casarin C, Cechotto A, Realdi R, Ruol A. Early detection of hepatocellular carcinoma in patients with cirrhosis by alphafetoprotein, ultrasound and fine-feedle biopsy. Hepatogastroenterology. 1989;35:519.
14. Bast, Th. Computertomographische Bildanalysen der Oberbauchorgane bei Thorotrastose und thorotrastinduzierten malignen Lebertumoren im computertomographischen und sonographischen Bild [Dissertation]. Heidelberg: University of Heidelberg; 1993.
15. Martinez A, Sánchez M, Roseló R. Selzer R, Alonso C, de Andrés L. Ultrasonic patterns observed in hepatic metastases from breast carcinoma: diagnosis and evolution. Gastrointest Radiol. 1989;14:49.
16. Beyer D, Schulze PJ. Sonographie der Leber. In: Bücheler E, Friedmann G, Thelen M, eds. Real-Time-Sonographie des Körpers. Stuttgart: Thieme; 1983.
17. Rubaltelli L, Maschio AD, Candiani F, Miotto D. The role of vascularization in the formation of echographic study. Br J Radiol. 1980;53:1166.
18. Marchal GJ, Tshibwabwa-Tumba EA, Oyen R, Pylyser K, Goddeeris R. Correlation of sonographic patterns in liver metastases with histology and microangiography. Invest Radiol. 1985;79:20.
19. Marchal GJ, Pylyser K, Tshibwabwa-Tumba EA, Verbeken E, Oyen R, Baert AL, Lauveryns JM. Anechoic halo in solid liver tumors: sonographic, microangiographic and histologic correlation. Radiology. 1985;156:479.
20. Wernecke K, Henke L, Vassallo P, Diederich S, Peters PE. Sonographic halo sign in liver tumors: histopathologic correlation. Radiology. 1991;181 (Suppl.):153.
21. Yoshida T, Matsue H. Okazaki N, Yoshimo M. Ultrasonographic differentiation of hepatocellular carcinoma from metastatic liver cancer. J Clin Ultrasound. 1987;15:431.
22. Wernecke K, Vasallo P, Bick U, Diederich S, Peters PE. Sonographic halo sign in liver tumors: clinical significance. Radiology. 1991;181 (Suppl.): 154.
23. Görich J, Kaick Gv. Sonographische Differentialdiagnostik herdfömiger Leberläsionen. Radiologe. 1988;28:349.
24. Wernecke K, Vassallo P, Bick U, Diederich S, Peters PE. The distinction between benign and malignant liver tumors on sonography: Value of a hypoechoic halo. Am J Roentgenol. 1992;159:1005.
25. Wernecke K, Peters PE. Sonographische und computertomographische Diagnostik von Lebermetastasen. Radiologe. 1985;25:141.
26. Schulz W, Hort W. The distribution of metastases in the liver – A quantitative postmortem study. Virchows Arch (A). 1981;394:89.
27. Wernecke K, Rummeny E, Bongartz G, Vassallo P, Kivelitz D, Wiesmann W, Peters PE, Rees B, Reiser M, Pircher W. Liver metastasis detection: comparative sensitivities of US, CT, and MR imaging for preoperative evaluation. Eur Radiol. 1991;1(Suppl.):169.
28. Wernecke K, Peters PE, Krüger K. Ultrasonographic patterns of focal hepatic and splenic lesions in Hodgkin's and non-Hodgkin's lymphoma. Br J Radiol 1987;60:655.
29. Schild H, Kreitner K, Thelen M, Grönninger J, Weber M, Börner N, Störkel J, Eißner D. Fokal-noduläre Hyperplasie der Leber bei 930 Patienten. Fortschr Röntgenstr. 1987;147:612.
30. Mathieu D, Bruneton JN, Drouillard J, Pointreau CC, Vasile N. Hepatic adenomas and focal nodular hyperplasia: dynamic CT study. Radiology. 1986;160:53.
31. Müller-Leisse C, Kujat C, Klose K, Büchsel R. Diagnostik der fokal-nodulären Hyperplasie. Röntgenpraxis. 1990; 43:281.
32. Lubbers PR, Ros PR, Goodman ZD, Ishak KG. Accumulation of technetium-99m sulfur colloid by hepatocellular adenoma—scintigraphic-pathologic correlation. Am J Roentgenol. 1986;148:1105.
33. Ashida C, Fishman EK, Zerhouni EA, Herlong FH, Siegelman SS. Computed tomography of hepatic cavernous hemangioma. J Comput Assist Tomogr. 1987;11:455.
34. Brodsky RI, Friedman AC, Maurer AH, Radecki PD, Caroline DF. Hepatic cavernous hemangioma: diagnosis with 99mTc labeled red cells and single-photon emission CT. Am J Roentgenol. 1987;148:125.
35. Engel MA, Marks DD, Sandler MA, Shetty P. Differentiation of local intrahepatic lesions with 99m-Tc red blood cell imaging. Radiology. 1983;146:777.
36. Lombardo DM, Baker ME, Spritzer CE, Blinder R, Meyers W, Herfkens RJ. Hepatic hemangiomas vs metastases: MR differentiation at 1.5 T. Am J Roentgenol. 1990;155:55.

37. Fobbe F, Hamm B, Schwarting R. Angiomyolipoma of the liver: CT, MR, and ultrasound imaging. J Comput Assist Tomogr. 1988;12:648.
38. Marti-Bonmati K, Menor F, Vizcaino I, Vilar J. Lipoma of the liver: US, CT, and MRT appearance. Gastrointest Radiol. 1989;14:155.
39. Brick SH, Hill MC, Lande IM. The mistake or indeterminate CT diagnosis of hepatic metastases: the value of sonography. Am J Roentgenol. 1987;148:723.
40. Swobodnik W, Wechsler JG, Manne W, Ditschuneit H. Multiple regular circumscript fatty infiltrations of the liver, J Clin Ultrasound. 1985;13:577.
41. Hess CF, Kurtz B, Grodd W, Wolf A. Hypoechoic lesions without halo in echogenic liver. Acta Radiol. 1989;29:541.
42. Haberkorn U, Zuna I, Lorenz A, Zerban H, Layer G, Kaick Gv, Räth U. Echographic tissue characterisation in diffuse parenchymal liver disease. Ultrasonic Imaging. 1990; 12:155.
43. Haberkorn U, Zuna I, Zerban H, Layer G, Lorenz A, Kaick Gv, Räth U. Quantitative Untersuchungen zum Einfluss von Bindegewebs- und Fettstrukturen auf das Ultraschallbild der Leber. Fortschr Röntgenstr. 1989;151:439.
44. Charnley RM, Morris DL, Dennison AR, Amar SS, Hardcastle JD. Detection of colorectal liver metastases using intraoperative ultrasonography. Br J Surg. 1991; 78:45.
45. Clarke MP, Kane RA, Steele G, Hamilton ES, Ravikumar TS, Onik G, Clouse ME. Prospective comparison of preoperative imaging and intraoperative ultrasonography in the detection of liver tumors. Surgery. 1988;106:849.
46. Hölscher AH, Stadler J. Intraoperative Sonographie zum Nachweis okkulter Lebermetastasen beim colorectalen Carcinom. Langenbecks Arch Chir. 1989;374:363.
47. Olsen AK. Intraoperative ultrasonography and the detection of liver metastases in patients with colorectal cancer. Br J Surg. 1990;77:998.
48. Börner NT, Clement T, Herzog P, Kreitner KF, Miltenberger H, Meyer J. Farbcodierte Dopplersonographic (FD-Sonographie) primärer und sekundärer Lebertumoren. Ultraschall Med. 1990;11:274.
49. Ohnishi K, Nomura F. Doppler studies of hepatocellular carcinoma and comparison with other hepatic focal lesions. Gastroenterology. 1990;97:1489.
50. Buscarini L, Formaro F, Bolondi L, Colombo P, Livraghi T, Magnolfi F, Rapaccini GL, Salmi A. Ultrasound-guided fineneedle biopsy of focal liver lesions: techniques. diagnostic accuracy and complications. J Hepatol. 1990;11:344.
51. Rettenmaier G. Fokale Leberveränderung. In: Rettenmaier G, Seitz K, eds. Sonographische Differentialdiagnostik. Weinheim: VCH; 1990.
52. Nelson RC, Chezmar JL. Diagnostic approach to hepatic hemangiomas. Radiology. 1990;176:11.

# 3

# SPIRAL CT OF THE LIVER

GREGORY T. SICA AND MARLA POLGER

The radiological evaluation of the liver using computed tomography (CT) has progressively evolved since its introduction in the early 1970s. This has been particularly true during the last decade. Numerous CT techniques have been described and are constantly being modified as the technology evolves. The ultimate goal is to attain the highest sensitivity and specificity for focal and diffuse liver disease using CT. This has become even more important with the advent of MR imaging as a competing modality for liver imaging.

It is generally believed that bolus contrast-enhanced rapid incremental scanning is currently the CT method of choice to image the liver. Using the dynamic incremental mode, 1–4-second single-slice axial images can be obtained serially with an inter-scan delay of 2–6 seconds. Using a 10-mm slice thickness allows the liver to be imaged within 2–3 minutes on average. A major drawback of this method is that spatial slice misregistration is likely to occur to some degree due to differences in the phase of respiration. Smaller lesions can be obscured by this effect, and multiplanar reformations can be adversely effected. In addition, scan time is prolonged by repeated respirations[1].

With regard to contrast enhancement, both monophasic and biphasic protocols have been advocated. Hepatic enhancement undergoes three phases: bolus, non-equilibrium and equilibrium. The basic objective is to scan the liver when liver-to-lesion contrast is maximum. This is best achieved when scanning occurs during the bolus and early non-equilibrium phases[2–4]. It has also been established that the greater the peak hepatic enhancement, the better lesion conspicuity will be[4–6]. Peak hepatic enhancement occurs during the first half of the non-equilibrium phase and can be increased by either increasing the contrast load or reducing the injection time[4,7,8]. Peak hepatic enhancement is greater and is achieved sooner by using a monophasic protocol than with a biphasic approach. A drawback, though, of the monophasic method is that the equilibrium phase of enhancement is also reached more quickly, thus allowing less time optimally to scan the liver. This knowledge has directed research efforts to devise new means for scanning the liver.

The development of slipring technology allowed the continuous acquisition of data over multiple 360-degree scans. This combined with continuous translation of the table mechanism through the gantry generates data in the shape of a helix. Using the filtered back projection method, axial images can then be reconstructed. Spiral or helical CT was introduced into general use in 1989 and represented an advance in rapid scanning. Since then, numerous reports have been published describing its use in imaging the liver, pancreas, kidneys, chest, head, neck and vascular system.

Spiral CT offers several advantages over conventional CT in imaging the liver. The primary advantage is the ability to perform single breath hold volume data acquisition, thus eliminating respiratory and motion artifacts, and ensuring section-to-section contiguity. Small lesions are thus less likely to be

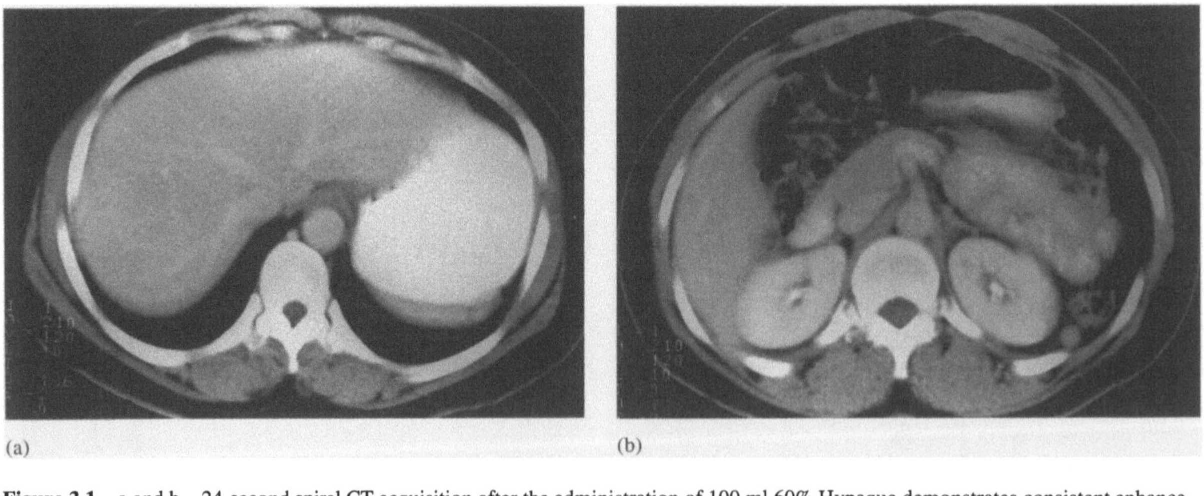

(a) (b)

**Figure 3.1** a and b 24-second spiral CT acquisition after the administration of 100 ml 60% Hypaque demonstrates consistent enhancement through the entire scan of the liver

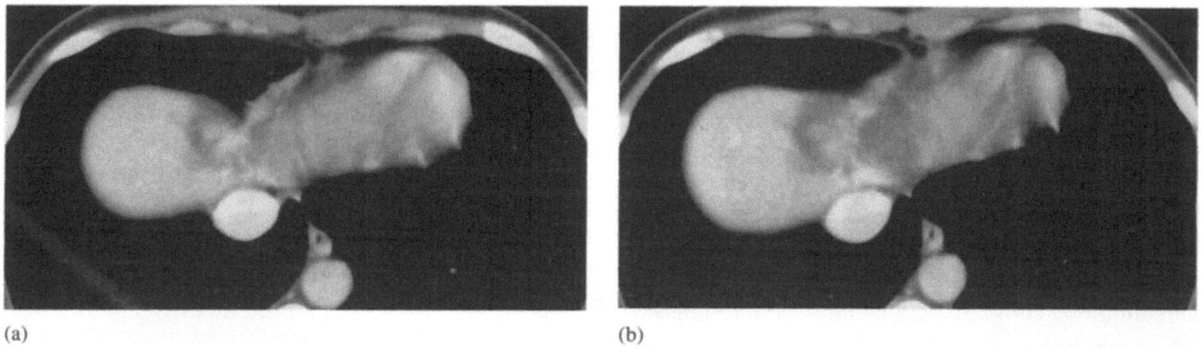

**Figure 3.2** a and b Targeted 24-second spiral acquisition of the liver dome region using 5 mm/s table feed speed, 5-mm collimation and 3-mm reconstruction increment. The study depicts a haemangioma in a location often difficult to image completely with conventional CT due to respiratory misregistration

missed. Three-dimensional reconstruction of hepatic anatomy, including vasculature, can be performed more reliably. As scanning time is shorter with spiral CT, the entire liver can be imaged during the non-equilibrium phase of a contrast-enhanced study. This optimizes the use of intravenous contrast and may ultimately allow a reduction in the volume of contrast used. Finally, lesion densitometry can be accurate because of the ability retrospectively to reconstruct axial images at any level within the volume data set[9-11].

Spiral scanning places a significant burden on the X-ray generators and tubes, although this has not been the limiting factor in tube design. Anode heat accumulation has been a more difficult feature to overcome[12]. The rate of anode heat dissipation limits the maximum mAs for a given length of spiral exposure, ultimately limiting the volume of tissue that can be scanned per single spiral. This limitation has been somewhat overcome by the production of more efficient X-ray detectors and X-ray tubes with a higher heat capacity.

Another significant disadvantage of spiral CT is volume averaging artifacts which result from an increase in the full width at half maximum (FWHM) with broadening of the section sensitivity slice profiles, particularly at the tails. Due to table motion during data acquisition, the shape of this curve assumes a more gaussian form with spiral CT rather than the rectangular shape seen with conventional CT. This effect is most notable in structures which change shape in the longitudinal direction (e.g. kidney) and

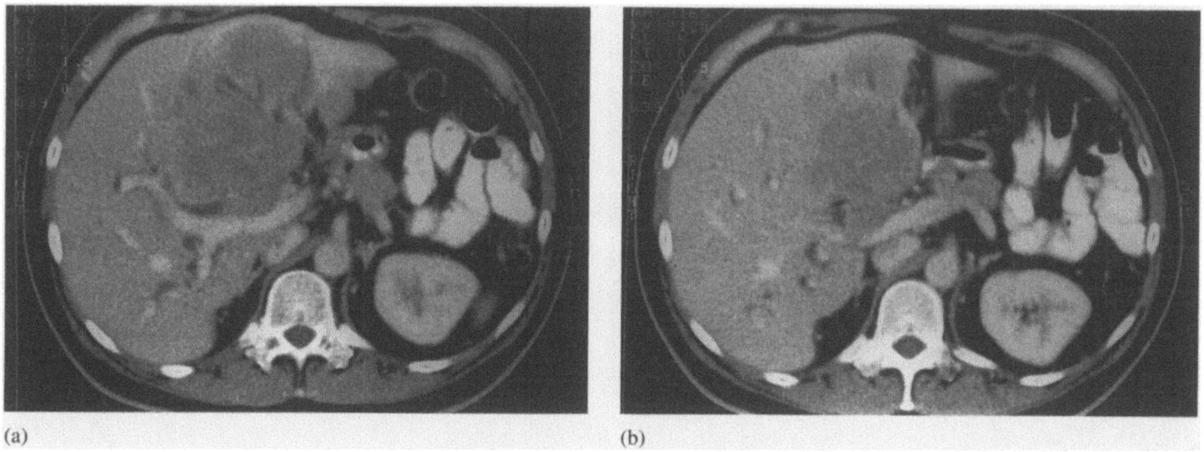

**Figure 3.3** a and b 24-second spiral CT acquisition of the liver after the administration of 100 ml 60% Hypaque demonstrates a hepatocellular carcinoma in the left lobe of the liver with portal vein invasion and billary ductal dilatation

results in blurring or irregularity of borders[13]. This may be partly overcome by decreasing slice thickness[3,9]. In addition, reconstruction algorithms have recently been modified to reduce this effect[11,12].

Other imaging parameters, such as spatial resolution in the imaging plane, image uniformity and contrast are unchanged when compared with conventional CT[13]. At a given mAs, pixel noise is decreased as planar data are interpolated from continuous raw data, including that above and below the scanning plane[1,9]. Radiation dose to the patient is unchanged compared with conventional methods if one chooses a table feed equal to the slice thickness[1]. In fact, the radiation dose may be less due to factors such as the inherently lower mA values and removing the need for overlapping images as in some conventional CT protocols or repeat imaging due to motion[13].

Several studies in the past few years have demonstrated the utility of spiral CT in imaging the liver. Zwicker et al.[14] reported identifying additional tumour nodules in six of 22 patients with hepatocellular carcinoma using spiral CT. In that study, images obtained with 10 mm collimation (table feed of 10 mm/s) were reconstructed at 5 mm and compared with conventional incremental dynamic CT. In addition, 35 hypervascular tumours were shown to be hyperattenuating with spiral CT but hypoattenuating with conventional CT. Urban et al.[10] compared 4-mm reconstruction with 8-mm using a table feed speed of 8 mm/s and 8-mm collimation. With a 4-mm reconstruction, 7% more lesions were detected in total, but 22% more were definitively identified. This represents a significant increase in confidence in detecting lesions. Bluemke et al.[15] reported the use of spiral CT with arterial portography. They conclude that high levels of parenchymal enhancement can be reliably obtained. This, combined with the lack of respiratory motion, allows the capability for quality three-dimensional reconstructions which may be useful in preoperative surgical planning.

Studies currently underway at Brigham and Women's Hospital[16], seek to assess the magnitude of contrast agent dose reduction for the liver that can be achieved without sacrificing hepatic enhancement. A prospective, randomized study was performed comparing various enhancement parameters amongst patients undergoing spiral and dynamic hepatic CT. The control group received 150 ml diatrizoate meglumine at a monophasic injection rate of 2.5 ml/s. The dynamic CT technique consisted of 1-s exposure amounting to a 6.5-s cycle time. The experimental groups received 75, 100 or 150 ml diatrizoate meglumine at the same monophasic injection rate of 2.5 ml/s. The delay for both the 150 ml control and experimental groups was 60 s, while the delay for the 75 and 100 ml experimental groups ranged from 30 to 60 s. The spiral CT technique for the experimental group consisted of a 24-s exposure, 10 mm/s table feed speed, and 10-mm slice collimation.

In the experimental groups, there was a linear dose–response relationship among the enhancements achieved for the three dosages that was statistically significant ($p < 0.0001$)[16]. Comparing the 150 ml spiral and dynamic groups, both the peak and average

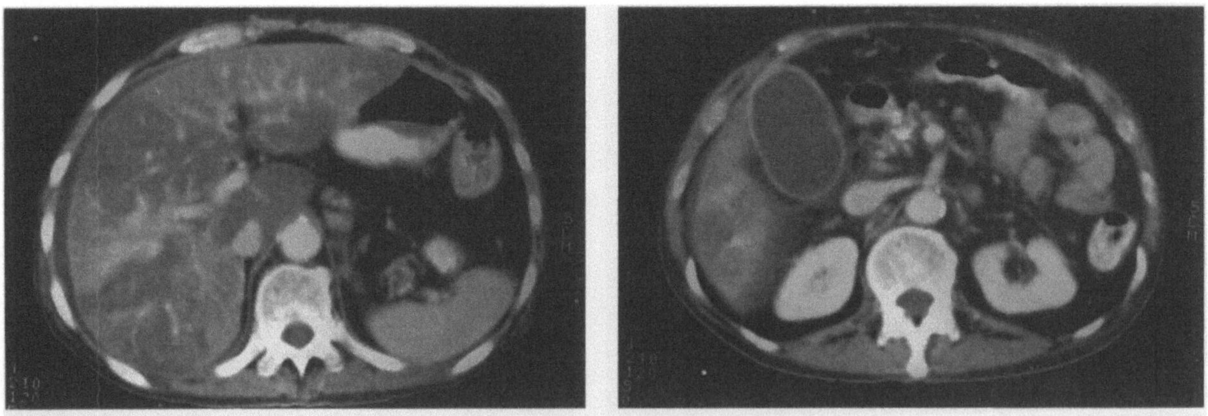

(a) (b)

**Figure 3.4** a and b 24-second spiral CT acquisition of the liver after the administration of 100 ml 60% Hypaque demonstrates geographic fatty infiltration liver enhancement values were higher with spiral CT, though this was not statistically significant. However, the enhancement on the last slice of liver was significantly different ($p = 0.011$)[17]. Using the spiral technique, a 30% dose reduction would be predicted to result in the same last slice enhancement achieved with a 150- ml dose and dynamic technique. As the caudal aspect of the liver is most apt to be imaged during the equilibrium phase with dynamic technique, this advantage of spiral CT may be particularly useful. A recent study showed that the use faster injection rates (5.0 ml/s) increased hepatic enhancement on dynamic CT[18]. Future investigations may show the benefits of faster injection rates to be even more substantial for spiral CT. These studies may ultimately lead to substantial savings in cost and reduced side-effects for patients.

## *References*


1. Kalender WA, Seissler W, Klotz E, Vock P. Spiral volumetric CT with single-breath-hold technique, continuous transport, and continuous scanner rotation. Radiology. 1990; 176:181–3.
2. Burgener FA, Hamlin DJ. Contrast enhancement of hepatic tumors in CT: Comparison between bolus and infusion techniques. Am J Roentgenol. 1983;140:291–5.
3. Burgener FA, Hamlin DJ. Contrast enhancement in abdominal CT: Bolus versus infusion. Am J Roentgenol. 1981; 137:617–22.
4. Cox IH, Foley WD, Hoffmann RG. Right window for dynamic hepatic CT. Radiology. 1991:181:18–21.
5. Marchal GJ, Baert AL, Wilms GE. CT of noncystic liver lesions: Bolus-enhancement. Am J Roentgenol. 1980; 135:57–65.
6. Young SW, Turner RJ, Castellino RA. A strategy for the contrast enhancement of malignant tumors using dynamic computed tomography and intravascular pharmacokinetics. Radiology. 1980;137:137–47.
7. Berland LL, Lee JY. Comparison of contrast media injection rates and volumes for hepatic dynamic incremental computer tomography. Invest Radiol. 1988;23:918–22.
8. Dean PB, Violante MR, Mahoney BS. Hepatic CT contrast enhancement: Effect of dose, duration of infusion, and time elapsed following infusion. Invest Radiol. 1980;15:158–61.
9. Brink JA, Heiken JP, Balfe DM, Sagel SS, DiCroce J, Vannier MW. Spiral CT: decreased spatial resolution *in vivo* due to broadening of section-sensitivity profile. Radiology. 1992; 185:469–74.
10. Urban BA, Fishman EK, Kuhlman JE, Kawashima A, Hennessey JG, Siegelman SS. Detection of focal hepatic lesions with spiral CT: Comparison of 4- and 8- mm interscan spacing. Am J Roentgenol. 1993;160:783–5.
11. Polacin A, Kalender WA, Marchal G. Evaluation of section sensitivity profiles and image noise in spiral CT. Radiology. 1992;185:29–35.
12. Zeman RK, Fox SH, Silverman PM, Davros WJ, Carter LM, Griego D, Weltman DI, Ascher SM. Cooper CJ. Helical (spiral) CT of the abdomen. Am J Roentgenol. 1993; 160:719–25.
13. Kalender WA. Polacin A. Physical performance characteristics of spiral CT scanning. Med Phys. 1991;18:910–5.
14. Zwicker C, Larger MF, Langer R, Rosenkranz K, Keske U. Spiral CT of hypervascular liver tumors and liver transplants. Radiology. 1991;181(P):95.
15. Bluemke DA, Fishman EK. Spiral CT arterial portography of the liver. Radiology. 1993;186:576–9.
16. Polger M, Seltzer SE, Adams DF, Silverman SG. Impact of intravenous contrast agent dose reduction in spiral CT of the liver. Radiology. 1992;185(P:)110.
17. Polger M, Seltzer SE, Adams DF, Silverman SG, Savci G. Spiral CT of the liver: potential for improved hepatic enhancement. Acad Radiol. 1994; in press.
18. Heiken JP, Brink JA, McClennan BL, Sagel SS, Forman HP, DiCroce J. Dynamic contrast-enhanced CT of the liver: Comparison of contrast medium injection rates and uniphasic and biphasic injection protocols. Radiology. 1993; 187:327–31.

4

# IMAGING OF HEPATIC NEOPLASMS IN PATIENTS WITH DIFFUSE LIVER DISEASE

UDO P. SCHMIEDL AND PATRICK C. FREENY

'Imagination is more important than knowledge'
A. Einstein

Finding and identifying hepatic neoplasms in patients with diffuse liver disease is one of the most challenging tasks in diagnostic radiology. This chapter discusses the performance of contrast enhanced CT (CECT), delayed iodine CT scan (DIS), magnetic resonance imaging (MR) and ultrasound (US) in detection and characterization of focal liver lesions in patients with diffuse liver disease. First, the sensitivity and specificity of these various imaging modalities for detection of focal lesions in patients with normal liver parenchyma is summarized. In the second part, the impact of diffuse liver disease on lesion detection is outlined. Finally, future strategies for the use of contrast agents targeted to liver in patients with diffuse liver disease are outlined.

## Hepatic imaging modalities

A variety imaging modalities is available to evaluate patients with suspected or known focal lesions of the liver. Consequently, a large number of studies has been published comparing the sensitivity of these imaging modalities, with respect to identifying the specific number of individual liver lesions, as well as to detecting patients with focal liver lesions. These studies have described a wide range of sensitivities, owing in part to limited pathological correlation, retrospective study design, differences in technique, and biased patient selection. Nevertheless, the studies have demonstrated that the overall sensitivity of imaging techniques, with the exception of CT angiography (CTA) and CT portography (CTAP), is limited with respect to tumour nodule detection, but is somewhat better with respect to detection of patients who have one or more focal lesions.

Three questions must be considered when comparing the diagnostic performance of cross-sectional hepatic imaging modalities:

1. The sensitivity for detection of tumour nodules;
2. The sensitivity for identifying patients with one or more focal liver lesions; and
3. Performance of the modality under investigation regarding the two prior questions in the setting of diffuse liver disease, most commonly liver cirrhosis.

Most studies that have compared the sensitivity for the detection of focal liver lesions have been performed in patients with at least a priori normal liver parenchyma. The sensitivity for the detection of focal liver lesions with CECT has been reported to be as low 38%[1] and as high as 90%[2]. The sensitivities of CTAP and CTA have been shown to range between 77% and 94%[3,4] and are generally considered the modalities of choice for preoperative evaluation of patients with metastatic liver disease who are potential candidates for hepatic resection.

Conventional MR imaging without the use of intravenous contrast has been shown to be between 63%[5] and 91%[2] sensitive for the detection of focal liver lesions. The sensitivity of CECT for identifying patients with hepatic neoplasms has been reported to be as low as 72%[5] and as high as 91%[2]. MR sensitivities for the identification of patients with liver lesions have been shown to range between 55%[5] and 96%[2].

A study reported in 1990 showed the highest lesion detection rate with CTA and did not show improvement in lesion detection sensitivity when additional modalities were combined, including DIS and MR[6]. The detection rate of hepatic tumours with different imaging techniques has thus been reported to be highly variable between different techniques and between different investigators studying identical techniques (Table 4.1). Inherent limitations of such studies, such as small patient population, limited pathological correlation, retrospective studies, or biased patient selection, may explain the large variability.

## Hepatic imaging and diffuse liver disease

Most studies have addressed finding nodules in livers with normal or at least relatively normal function. Only a few studies with gross pathological validation have attempted to measure the sensitivity of imaging studies to detect focal lesions in livers with diffuse changes, in particular cirrhosis. Diffuse changes in the liver parenchyma are often encountered in daily clinical practice. Disease entities that are summarized under the term 'diffuse liver disease' comprise cirrhosis, hepatic iron overload and fatty infiltration. Less commonly, copper deposition, glycogen storage disease, sarcoidosis, and vascular pathology, such as Budd Chiari syndrome, can lead to diffuse changes of the liver parenchyma. Liver fibrosis, either diffuse

**Table 4.1 Detection of tumour nodules**

| *Author* | *CT* | *DIS* | *CTA(AP)* | *MR* |
|---|---|---|---|---|
| Freeny and Ryan[6] | 55% | 70% | 80% | 64% |
| Heiken et al.[1] | 38% | | 81% | 57% |
| Bernardino[2] | 70% | 71% | | 77% |
| Nelson[56] | | 66% | 85% | 69% |
| Sitzman et al.[4] | 66% | | 94% | 70% |
| Wernecke et al.[5] | 67% | | | 63% |
| **Total** | 59% | 72% | 84% | 69% |

congenital hepatic fibrosis, or posthepatitic or alcoholic fibrosis, produces changes in the liver architecture and extrahepatic changes that are readily detected by CECT.

The presence of diffuse liver disease is usually detected by means of laboratory and histological techniques, and imaging techniques play a secondary role. In some instances, diffuse liver disease is discovered by chance during a diagnostic imaging test performed for other reasons.

Although the issue of detection and staging of hepatic metastasis arises in patients with diffuse liver disease, the more common question the radiologist is confronted with is the detection of hepatocellular carcinomas in patients with cirrhosis. Patients with diffuse liver disease, in particular cirrhosis, are at much greater risk of developing primary malignant tumours of the liver compared with the general population. If detected early, surgery, including resection or transplantation, offers the only cure. The early detection of these tumours is heavily dependent on the imaging techniques. Since diffuse liver disease changes the architecture of the liver parenchyma and can also have focal manifestations, it is helpful to understand the manifestations of diffuse liver disease as seen with modern imaging modalities (Figure 4.1). The discussion will focus mainly on image manifestations of fatty infiltration, cirrhosis, and iron overload. These conditions frequently occur in the setting of abnormal size, shape or contour of the liver associated with heterogeneous parenchymal attenuation values, signal intensity or echogenicity.

## Fatty infiltration

Fatty infiltration of the liver is caused by increased deposition of triglycerides within hepatocytes. This occurs in various conditions, such as chronic alcoholism, intravenous or oral hyperalimentation, Cushing's disease or corticosteroid therapy, diabetes mellitus, post-jejuno-ileal bypass, Reye's syndrome, kwashiorkor, and betalipoproteinaemia. Patients with advanced malignancies commonly have fatty livers secondary to chemotherapy and poor nutrition. In some cases, particularly in patients with Cushing's disease, corticosteroid therapy, early diabetes mellitus or obesity, deposition of fat in the liver can result in a homogeneous or heterogeneous distribution. Patchy or even focal fatty changes probably reflect regional differences in hepatic perfusion. Areas with decreased portal flow tend to accumulate less fat than better-perfused areas[7,8]. Regional fatty infiltration may also occur in areas with better portal perfusion.

Attenuation values of liver in normal patients show a wide distribution[9]. Thus a low mean attenuation value may be misleading. However, comparison of liver and spleen density often allows one to determine the presence of fatty liver. Fatty infiltration caused by alcoholism and intravenous hyperalimentation frequently produces a heterogeneous appearance. In patients with long-standing diabetes, the distribution of fat is also extremely variable. Occasionally, localized collections of fat may produce the appearance of focal or multifocal lesions, thus suggesting either a primary tumour or metastases. Typically, normal hepatic vessels can be seen to course through these areas of low density and the correct diagnosis of focal fat can be made. On CT images, metastases may be isodense with fatty liver, eluding detection[10]. Other imaging characteristics of focal fatty liver or focal sparing include a wedge-shaped area of different attenuation or signal intensity and lack of mass effect. However, these findings are absent in many patients. Small regions of fatty liver may be espe-

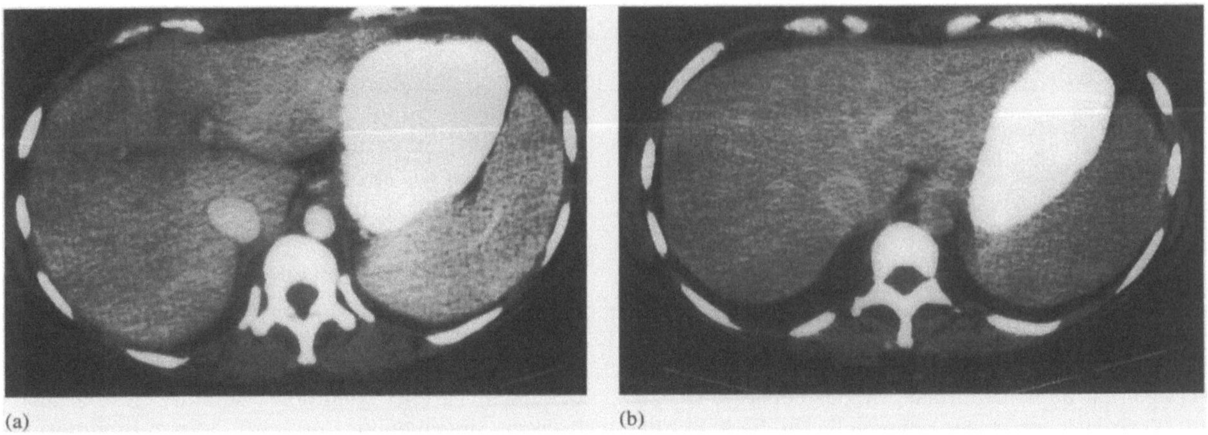

**Figure 4.1** a. CECT shows an ill-defined low-attenuation area in the medial segment of the left lobe and the anterior segment of the right lobe of the liver. b. DIS at the same level as (a) shows homogeneous attenuation of the liver. No focal lesion was found in this patient with cryptogenic cirrhosis. The low-attenuation area presumably represents a perfusion defect

cially difficult to distinguish from malignant lesions, since small tumours do not show mass effect or obvious exclusion of hepatic vessels. Thus, diagnosis of focal hepatic lesions may often be difficult in patients with fatty infiltration.

Certain regions of the liver commonly have fatty infiltration, such as the medial segment of the left lobe adjacent to the falciform ligament[11]. The area of the medial segment adjacent to the portal vein and the caudate lobe, on the other hand, are commonly spared in a diffusely fatty liver[12].

Fatty infiltration of the liver has been shown, both in experimental animals and humans, to increase the liver signal intensity (SI) on T1 weighted MR images. Proton spectroscopic imaging has also been used to determine the fat content of the liver[13]. More commonly, however, SI of liver parenchyma is unchanged in patients with fatty infiltration.

MR techniques that rely on the different resonances of water and fat protons can also assist in differentiating focal fat from other liver lesions. Chemical shift imaging allows diagnosis of fatty hepatic abnormalities in instances where focal or diffuse fatty infiltration of the liver is considered in the differential diagnosis. Opposed phase imaging or fat saturation techniques are also very effective for detecting fatty liver[14]. By comparing T1 weighted spin echo images with fat-suppressed or opposed phase images, differentiation between focal fat and neoplasms should be possible. Fatty areas should have a higher signal on T1 weighted images with expected signal drop with fat-suppressed techniques. Metastases typically have a low SI on T1 weighted images and they do not demonstrate relative decrease in SI with fat-suppression techniques. This concept has to be modified when examining a liver with a possible hepatocellular carcinoma, adenoma, focal nodular hyperplasia, regenerative nodule or lipomatous tumours. These masses may contain variable amounts of fat, melanin, copper, iron or blood products which can result in a high SI on T1 weighted images. Chemical shift imaging should allow distinction between masses containing melanin or blood products. A hepatocellular carcinoma contains fat that is typically is well differentiated and defined, often has a capsule and contains some other material that has a high SI on T2 weighted images[15,16].

Echogenicity depends on the amount of fat deposition and the number of droplets. The echogenicity of fatty livers is generally increased on US. Areas of focal sparing in diffuse fatty infiltration are hypoechoic relative to the fatty liver. Areas that contain deposits of larger intracellular lipid droplets can also result in decreased echogenicity[17].

## Cirrhosis

The basic pathological process characterizing alcoholic, nutritional and posthepatitic cirrhosis is that of extensive collagen deposition, periportal and bridging fibrosis, and distortion of the normal hepatic lobular architecture[18]. CT may not show any abnormality in patients with cirrhosis. More commonly, however, liver changes are identifiable that include decrease in overall size, nodular contour, enlargement of the caudate lobe, and heterogeneous parenchyma[19] (Figure 4.1). Fatty infiltration, which is relatively rare in cirrhosis, is demonstrated by a mixture of low-density areas irregularly interspersed with areas of fibrosis and nodular regeneration. On occasion, a diffusely enlarged liver that has a homogeneously decreased density may be seen. Iron deposition also occurs in cirrhotic livers, decreasing the liver SI on T2 weighted images. Portal hypertension is a secondary sign of cirrhosis and is characterized by splenomegaly, varices and a recanalized umbilical vein.

A prospective study identified a correlation between the ratio of MR SI of liver and fat and on short inversion-recovery images (STIR)[20]. Patients with severe chronic liver disease had brighter liver SI than those with less severe disease. Significant differences were found between signal intensities of normal livers and those of diseased livers, of which the latter were brighter than normal livers on STIR images. It was believed that the increased signal was due to periportal and lobular necrosis and portal inflammation. While fibrosis may not significantly alter the signal characteristics of the liver on conventional T1 and T2 weighted spin echo images[13], it has been postulated that hepatitis changes the signal intensity[21]. Experimental studies have demonstrated increased relaxation times occurring within a short period of time following the induction of hepatitis, owing to the relatively increased water content of the inflamed liver[22].

The detection of liver cirrhosis by US has received limited attention in the recent imaging literature. Typically, cirrhosis is manifested by greatly increased beam attenuation compared with normal liver. In addition, changes in size and contour of the liver can be detected. The liver is often seen as enlarged, or shrunken and lobulated with increased echogenicity and a coarse echotexture. The use of relative measurements of the liver lobes has been suggested to establish the diagnosis of liver cirrhosis[23–25]. The diagnosis of cirrhosis by means of surface changes has been proposed but the limitations of this approach are recognized[26,27]. Duplex and colour Doppler are used routinely to assess the inter- and extrahepatic vascular changes associated with cirrhosis. Hepatic echogenicity is also increased in patients with haemochromatosis and diffuse metastatic disease. Thus, many processes can result in altered echogenicity of the liver and they cannot be differentiated based on the US appearance. The diagnosis of diffuse liver disease by US therefore ambiguous.

**Focal lesions in cirrhotic livers**

Regenerative nodules result from grossly distorted hepatic architecture, heterogeneous regeneration of liver parenchyma, and hepatocellular dysplasia. Regenerating nodules are common in cirrhosis and appear as focal masses that have CT attenuation values similar to normal liver parenchyma (Figure 4.2). Bands of fibrosis usually surround the regenerating nodules[28]. The amount of fibrosis in a lobe may vary from one area to another and may vary between lobes. Areas of fibrosis without regenerating nodules can appear as a focal lesions[25,29]. Although areas of massive fibrosis have been reported to exhibit characteristic CT features, including a wedge shape and peripheral location, they may be mistaken for hepatic neoplasms[29] (Figure 4.3).

Regenerative nodules larger than 5 mm have been found in 39% of cirrhotic livers and nodules larger than 10 mm have been found in approximately 11%[30–32] (Figure 4.4). These nodules are typically hypoechoic relative to cirrhotic liver on US, thus mimicking hepatocellular carcinoma (HCC). The sensitivity of US for the detection of these lesions is not well established. MR imaging can show regenerating nodules as low SI relative to high SI of inflamed fibrous septa or damaged liver[33]. Often, regenerating nodules are bright on T1 and dark T2 weighted images, helping to differentiate them from HCC, which can be bright or dark on T1, but are virtually always bright on T2. Some regenerating nodules may accumulate iron more than surrounding liver parenchyma, resulting in a relatively lower SI on T2 weighted images[34]. Some large nodules in cirrhotic livers have dysplastic histological characteristics including foci of dysplasia or malignancy, iron or fat accumulation[30,34,35]. HCC can mimic other focal lesions, such as regenerating nodules (Figures 4.5, 4.6 and 4.7). They can remain entirely undetected in cirrhotic livers despite use of several imaging modalities, including CECT, DIS, CAP and contrast enhanced MR (Figure 4.8).

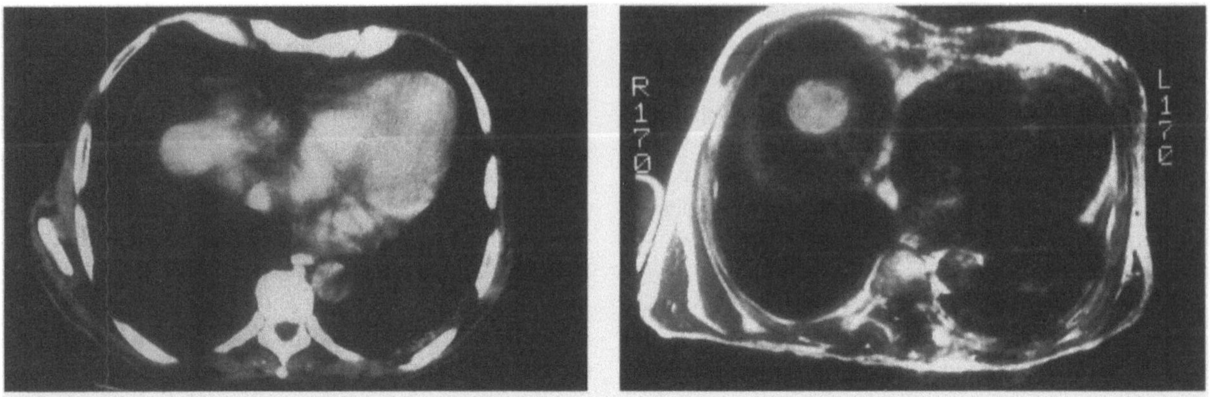


(a) (b)

**Figure 4.2** a. CECT demonstrates a well-defined mass at the dome of the liver. This patient was evaluated for liver transplantation. The mass is bright on the T1 weighted SE image (b) and had low SI on the T2 weighted image (not shown). A regenerating nodule was found at pathology following orthotopic liver transplantation

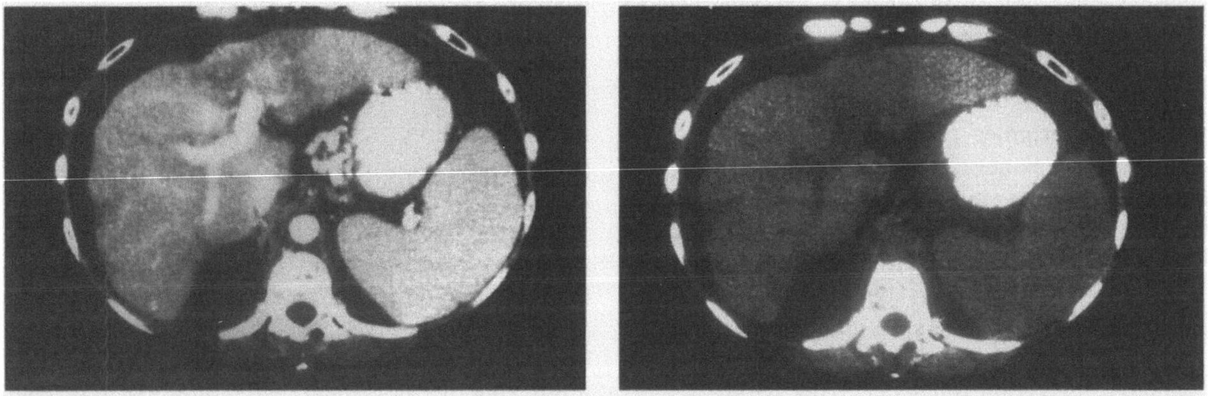

(a) (b)

**Figure 4.3** CECT (a) and DIS (b) in a patient with cirrhosis and portal hypertension (gastric varices and splenomegaly) show an ill-defined heterogeneous area in the left lobe of the liver. Pathological evaluation revealed confluent hepatic fibrosis without evidence for neoplasm

Segmental hepatic atrophy and compensatory hypertrophy can mimic hepatic masses. This can be caused by acute hepatitis, portal vein or biliary obstruction, sclerosing cholangitis, and end stage cirrhosis. Segmental atrophy may be manifested as a wedge-shaped region and, occasionally, atrophied liver may be seen as a focal mass with abnormal MR signal intensity.

It is important to detect and correctly classify large adenomatous hyperplastic (AH) nodules in cirrhotic livers, since these lesions, particularly if they accumulate fat or iron, have a greater malignant potential than other nodules[34]. Nodules should be carefully examined for internal foci that are typically bright on T2 weighted images. If a suspicious nodule is identified, a percutaneous biopsy may often yield equivocal results since many of the HCC which arise in these nodules are small and well differentiated. Serological markers for HCC, such as $\alpha$-fetoprotein, are usually normal in these patients.

SI differences and morphology may be helpful for differentiating between HCC and regenerative or AH nodules. AH nodules often have high SI on T1 weighted images and are iso or hypodense on T2 weighted images[36]. Most HCC have a high SI on T2 weighted images and can thus be differentiated from AH nodules. Well-differentiated HCC and fibrolamellar HCC have signal characteristics of

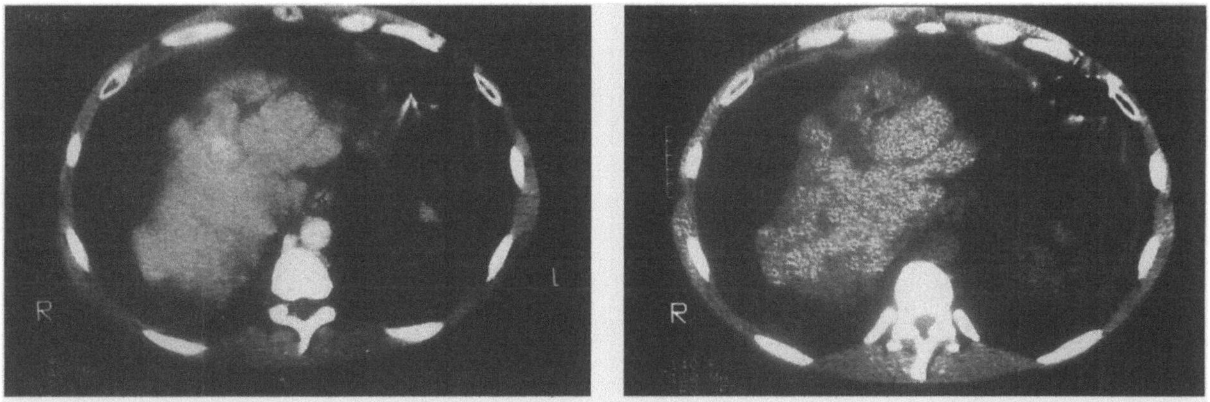


(a) (b)

**Figure 4.4** CECT (a) and DIS (b) shows multiple heterogeneous masses in this small liver. Pathology following liver transplantation revealed multiple regenerating nodules and liver cirrhosis. No neoplasm was found

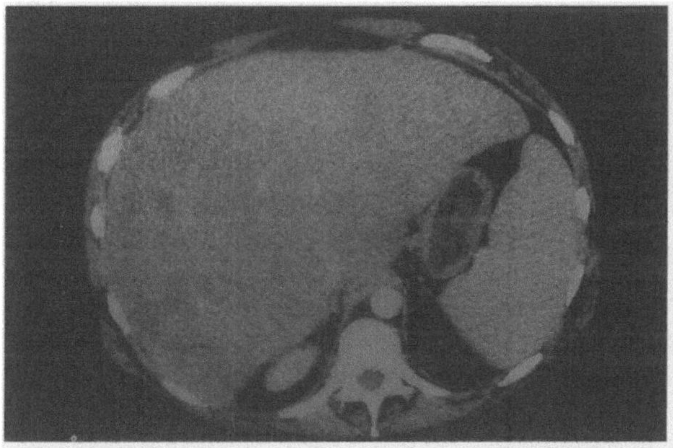

**Figure 4.5** CECT shows hepatosplenomegaly and ill-defined low-attenuation areas in this patient with a diffusely infiltrating hepatocellular carcinoma. CECT appearance is indistinguishable from the perfusion defect shown in Figure 1a

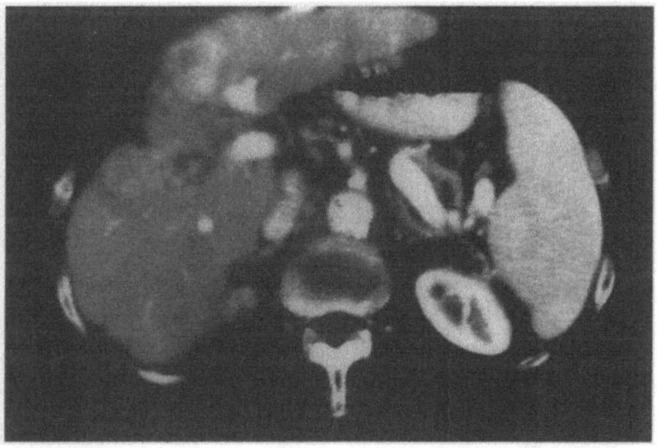

**Figure 4.6** CECT demonstrates a nodular contour of the liver and a heterogeneous area in the left lobe of the liver. Thrombosis of the left portal vein and recanalization of the umbilical vein is present. Biopsy confirmed a hepatocellular carcinoma in the left lobe that had invaded the left portal vein

hyperplastic nodules, consistent with the histological similarity between these two lesions[16,37]. CT contrast enhancement patterns may differ between benign and malignant nodules. AH nodules are primarily supplied by the portal vein, while HCC are supplied almost exclusively by the hepatic artery. Thus, AH nodules are expected to enhance in a similar fashion to liver parenchyma, while HCC usually enhances less than surrounding liver during the early portal phase following bolus contrast administration[38,39]. CTAP may even be more reliable for differentiation[40]. Overlapping patterns have been documented, however. Well-differentiated HCC often retains some portal perfusion, and benign AH nodules may have increased arterial perfusion. Furthermore, enhancement patterns in patients with cirrhosis may be even more confusing owing to overall decreased portal perfusion and increased hepatic arterial perfusion.

Detection of focal liver lesions in the setting of diffuse lever disease by US is limited by the altered beam penetration, difficulty in diagnosing liver cirrhosis, and the occurrence of regenerating nodules which may mimic primary or secondary neoplasms. Even when the presence of cirrhosis had been established, only 50% of patients that had malignant neoplasms were identified by US[41]. In another study with pathological correlation, US showed only 36

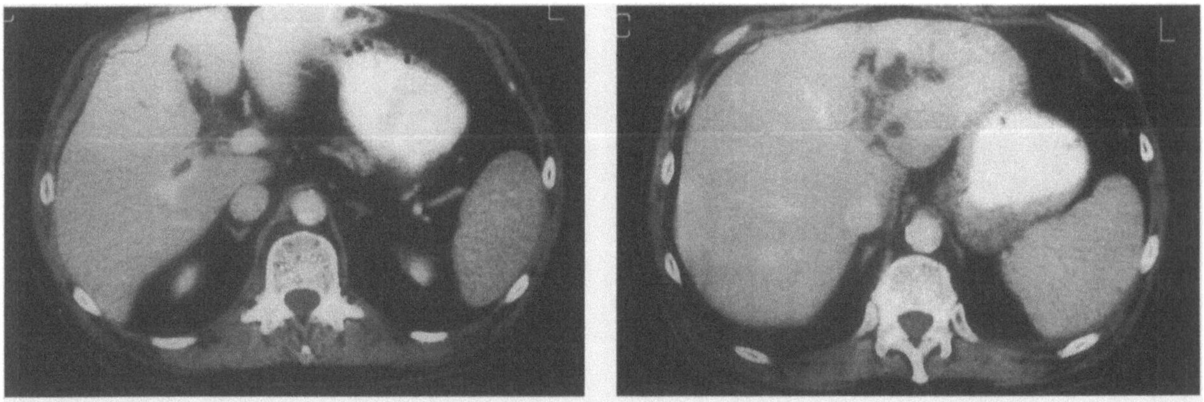

(a) (b)

**Figure 4.7** a and b CECT at two levels shows a low-attenuation lesion in the lateral segment of the left lobe. Thrombus is present in the left and posterior right portal vein. This patient had a liver abscess with septic thrombosis of the portal vein secondary to diverticulitis

of 80 HCC lesions, resulting in a sensitivity of 45%[42].

Thus, imaging characteristics of a variety of masses overlap and specific diagnosis of lesions is often not possible based on imaging findings alone.

## Haemochromatosis and glycogen storage disease

Haemochromatosis and glycogen storage disease produce increased liver density on CT. Iron deposition in the liver may either occur in the hepatocytes

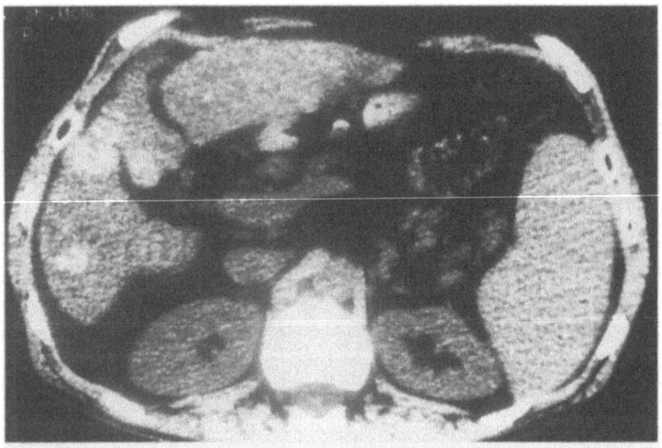

(a)

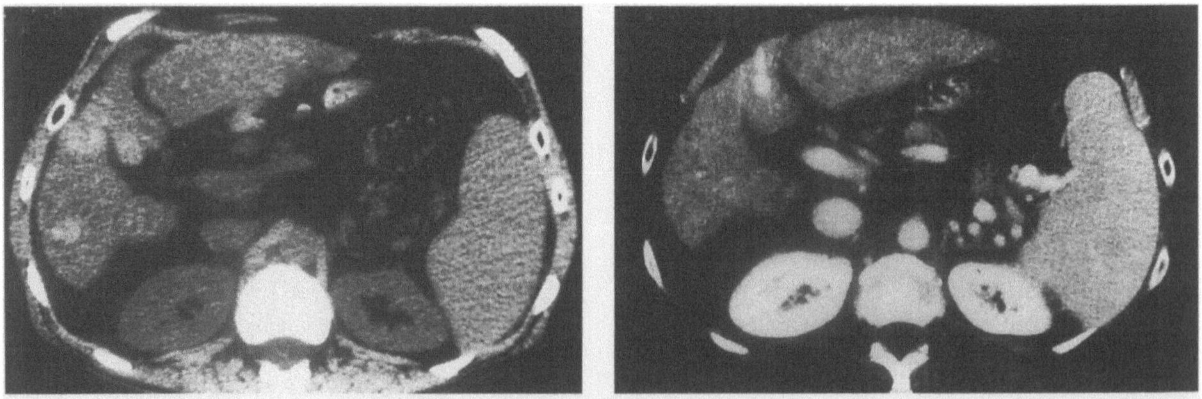

(b) (c)

**Figure 4.8** CTAP (a) and DIS (b) showed hyperdense lesions in the right lobe of the liver in a patient being evaluated for liver transplantation. CECT (c) showed heterogeneity of the right lobe. The left lobe was unremarkable on every CT scan. Also MR scans, including Gd-enhanced T1 weighted images, showed a normal left lobe. Following liver transplantation, a 3-cm hepatocellular carcinoma was found in the left lobe of the liver, undetected by all imaging modalities. The lesions in the right lobe proved to be regenerating nodules (haemochromatosis) or in the Kupffer (reticuloendothelial) cells. Haemochromatosis involves increased iron absorption and iron deposition in hepatocytes, pancreas, heart, and other organs. Iron deposition which occurs in the reticuloendothelial cells will also affect the spleen, lymph nodes, and pancreas, and, in later stages, the myocardium. This may be either a primary process or secondary to breakdown of red blood cells owing to congenital haemolytic anaemias or transfusions.

Hepatic MR signal in patients with increased iron deposition is decreased owing to increased bulk susceptibility which reduces T2* relaxation time. Normal liver is isointense or slightly more intense relative to skeletal muscle on virtually all pulse sequences and skeletal muscle is unaffected in patients with iron overload. Thus, skeletal muscle can be used as a reference tissue for quantitating decreased hepatic signal intensity[43].

Cirrhosis and hepatocellular carcinomas are common in patients with haemochromatosis. Tumour cells typically do not contain excessive iron: thus they have a high liver-to-lesion contrast in livers with iron overload. Livers demonstrate high attenuation on precontrast CT scans. Administration of contrast may decrease lesion-to-liver contrast because of high baseline attenuation values of liver parenchyma and rapid equilibration between tumour and liver.

## Role and limitations of contrast media

As already indicated above, diffuse liver disease will decrease the sensitivity of any imaging modality in detection of focal liver lesions. In addition, there are focal manifestations of diffuse liver disease that can be confused with hepatic neoplasms.

Intravenous contrast material causes other obstacles for the detection of focal hepatic tumours in patients with diffuse liver disease, particularly cirrhosis. Heterogeneous hepatic enhancement patterns in diffuse liver disease may mimic neoplastic lesions and thus result in false positive diagnoses. Secondly, heterogeneous attenuation of SI in diffuse liver disease changes the lesion-to-liver contrast on both pre- and postcontrast images, significantly impairing visibility of lesions. Thirdly, vascular perfusion patterns in cirrhotic livers are altered. Even if the intrahepatic portal system is largely patent in patients with cirrhosis, diffuse changes of the hepatic architecture cause heterogeneous distribution of blood flow and heterogeneous parenchymal enhancement. Alternatively, cirrhotic liver parenchyma may show increased CT or MR enhancement during dynamic or equilibrium phases after administration of intravenous contrast. One possible explanation for this increased enhancement is the relative increase in hepatic arterial perfusion in areas of decreased portal blood flow. Thus, enhancement patterns and enhancement levels seen in patients with normal livers often cannot be achieved in patients with cirrhosis. This makes the detection of liver lesions even more challenging given the already increased heterogeneity of the cirrhotic liver on precontrast scans.

Most of the experience in using contrast material for liver imaging has been with extracellular fluid contrast agents, in particular iodinated contrast agents for CT and small molecular weight chelates for MR. The fundamental limitation of these contrast agents is their delivery to tumours via the hepatic artery before contrast material reaches normal liver via the portal circulation and rapid equilibration of the contrast material between intravascular and extracellular fluid space in both normal liver and tumours. These limitations are compounded in patients with liver disease owing to alterations of the hepatic architecture and perfusion.

Iodinated contrast material has been encapsulated in liposomes to improve hepatic enhancement. Intravenously injected iodinated liposomes are taken up by the reticuloendothelial system (RES) and persistently enhance normal liver parenchyma[44]. Experience with these agents in patients with liver disease has not been reported to date. Iodized oil droplets targeted to the RES have also undergone clinical trials as CT contrast agents[45].

A variety of MR contrast agents targeted to the liver is being investigated and two general strategies are being pursued. One strategy is to target the hepatocytes with either relatively lipophilic agents, such as Gd-EOB-DTPA or Gd-BOPTA, or manganese or iron chelates exhibiting hepatobiliary affinity[46–50]. The second strategy is to target the RES, specifically the Kupffer cells located on the surface of the vascular endothelium of the liver using coated iron particles[51]. While iron particles have mostly been used to decrease SI of normal liver parenchyma on T2 weighted studies, hepatocyte-directed agents have been used primarily to increase the SI of liver parenchyma. To date, it remains unclear which of the two alternatives will be advantageous in patients with diffuse liver disease. Impaired hepatic blood flow may alter the distribution pattern of any of these agents, thus influencing their diagnostic performance. Altered hepatocellular function may decrease hepatic uptake of agents that undergo hepatobiliary excretion and therefore result in decreased enhancement levels. Thus, these agents may not only be less efficacious in patients with decreased liver function, but they may also be contraindicated if they are mostly excreted through the hepatobiliary system. Furthermore, as outlined above, well-differentiated hepatic neoplasms retain some hepatocellular and reticuloendothelial function and are known to accumulate lipids and other intracellular material. It is not surprising, therefore, that in initial clinical studies, enhancement of HCC has been observed using the hepatocellular marker, Mn-DPDP[47]. While this may interfere with the detectability of HCC on enhanced scans, this feature may be useful to differentiate HCC from haemangioma, an occasional clinical problem.

Relatively low precontrast SI in cirrhotic livers with increased iron stores may narrow the enhancement yield using iron particles directed to the RES. Benign and malignant neoplasms may contain variable concentrations of Kupffer cells. Uptake of RES-directed agents would thus be expected in both tumour and liver parenchyma. This may interfere with lesion detectability and lesion characterization. Initial experience in animal models has indicated heterogeneous distribution of iron oxide in cirrhotic livers, potentially decreasing the diagnostic utility of this compound in the setting of diffuse liver disease[21].

Research into the use of contrast agents for US imaging is currently evolving. Most of the applications of US contrast agents have been in the area of vascular and perfusion imaging. While these agents may be useful for the improved detection of focal liver lesions, agents that are targeted to one of the major tissue components of the liver may be preferable[52–55].

The challenge for the future is to continue to design new agents targeted to the hepatobiliary system and to assess the diagnostic performance of the agents currently under investigation in the setting of diffuse liver disease. Cost-effective strategies will clearly have to be developed to utilize the imaging modalities at hand optimally to diagnose focal liver lesions in patients with diffuse liver disease.

## *References*


1. Heiken J, Weyman P, Lee J, et al. Detection of focal metastases: prospective evaluation with CT, delayed CT, CT during arterial portography, and MR imaging. Radiology. 1989; 171:47–51.
2. Bernardino M. Emory experience with both CT and MRI in the detection of focal liver disease. In: Ferruci J, Stark D, ed. Liver imaging. Current trends and new techniques. Boston: Andover Medical Publisher Inc.; 1990:73–81.
3. Miller D, Simmons J, Chang R, et al. Hepatic metastases: comparison of three CT contrast enhancement methods. Radiology. 1987;165:785–90.
4. Sitzman J, Coleman J, Pitt H, et al. Preoperative assessment of malignant hepatic tumors. Am J Surg. 1990;159:137–43.
5. Wernecke K, Rummeny E, Bongartz G, et al. Detection of hepatic masses in patients with carcinoma: comparative sensitivities of sonography, CT, and MR imaging. Am J Roentgenol. 1991;157:731–6
6. Freeny P, Ryan J. Preoperative hepatic imaging for lesion detection using bolus dynamic CT, CT angiography, delayed iodine CT, and MR. Presented at the 76th Assembly and Annual Meeting of the RSNA, Chicago, IL. November 25–30, 1990.
7. Arai K, Matsui O, Takashima T, et al. Focal spared areas in fatty liver caused by regional decreased portal flow. Am J Roentgenol. 1988;151:300–2.
8. Marchal G, Tschibwabwa-Tuma E, Verbeken E, et al. 'Skip areas' in hepatic steatosis: a sonographic–angiographic study. Gastrointest Radiol. 1989;11:151–7.
9. Pierkarski J, Goldberg HI, Royal SA, et al. Difference between liver and spleen CT numbers in the normal adult: its usefulness in predicting the presence of diffuse liver disease. Radiology. 1980; 137:727.
10. Lewis E, Bernardino ME, Barnes PA, et al. The fatty liver: pitfalls in the CT and angiographic evaluation of metastatic disease. J Comput Assist Tomogr. 1983;7:235–241.
11. Yoshikawa J, Matsui O, Takashima T, et al. Focal fatty change of the liver adjacent to the falciform ligament: CT and sonographic findings in 5 surgically confirmed cases. Am J Roentgenol. 1987;149:491–4.
12. Berland LL. Focal areas of decreased echogenicity in the liver at the porta hepatis. J Ultrasound Med. 1986; 5:157–9.
13. Goldberg HI, Margulis AR, Moss AA, et al. Imaging of the liver, gallbladder, spleen, pancreas, peritoneal cavity, and alimentary tube. In: James TL, Margulis AR, eds. Biomedical magnetic resonance, Chap 24. San Francisco: University of California; 1984.
14. Mitchell DM, Kim I, Chang TS, et al. Chemical shift phase difference and suppression magnetic resonance imaging techniques in animals, phantoms and humans: fatty liver. Invest Radiol. 1991;26:1041–52.
15. Itai Y, Ohtomo K, Kokubo T, et al. CT and MR imaging of fatty tumors of the liver. J. Comput Assist Tomogr. 1987; 11:253–7.
16. Ebara M, Watanabe S, Kita K, et al. MR imaging of small hepatocellular carcinoma: effect of intratumoral copper content on signal intensity. Radiology. 1991;180:617–21.
17. Caturelli E, Costarelli L, Giordano M, et al. Hypoechoic lesions in fatty liver: quantitative study by histomorphology. Gastroenterology. 1991;100:1678–82.
18. Popper H. Pathologic aspects of cirrhosis: a review. Am J Pathol. 1977;87:228–64.

19. Torres WE, Whitmire LF, McClees KG, Bernardino ME. Computed tomography of hepatic morphologic changes in cirrhosis of the liver. J Comput Assist Tomogr. 1986;10:47.
20. Marti-Bonmati L, Talens A, del Olmo J, et al. Chronic hepatitis and cirrhosis: evaluation by means of MR imaging with histologic correlation. Radiology. 1993;188:37–43.
21. Elizondo G, Weissleder R, Stark D, et al. Hepatic cirrhosis and hepatitis: MR imaging with superparamagnetic iron oxide. Radiology. 1990;174:797–801.
22. Stark D, Bass NM, Moss AA, et al. Nuclear magnetic imaging of experimentally induced liver disease. Radiology. 1983; 148:743.
23. Hess CF, Schmiedl U, Kölbel G, Knecht R, Kurtz B. US diagnosis of liver cirrhosis: ROC analysis of multidimensional caudate lobe indices. Radiology. 1989;171:349–51.
24. Goyal AK, Pokharna DS, Sharma SK. Ultrasonic diagnosis of cirrhosis. Reference to quantitave measurements of hepatic dimensions. Gastrointest Radiol. 1990;15:32–4.
25. Harbin WP, Robert NJ, Ferruci JT, Diagnosis of cirrhosis based on regional changes in hepatic morphology. A radiological analysis. Radiology. 1980;135:273.
26. Lelio AD, Cestari C, Lomazzi A, Beretta L. Cirrhosis: Diagnosis with sonographic study of the liver surface. Radiology. 1989;172:389–92.
27. Ladenheim JA, Luba G, Yao F, et al. Limitations of liver surface US in the diagnosis of cirrhosis. Radiology. 1992; 185:21–4.
28. Anthony PP, Ishak KG, Nayak NC, Poulsen HE, Scheuer PJ, Sobin LH. The morphology of cirrhosis. Recommendations on definition, nomenclature, and classification by a working group sponsored by the World Health Organization. J Clin Pathol. 1978;31:273–414.
29. Ohtomo K, Baron RL, Dodd GD, et al. Confluent hepatic fibrosis in advanced cirrhosis: diagnostic appearance on hepatic CT scans. Radiology. 1993;188:31–37.
30. Furuya K, Nakamura M, Yamamoto Y, et al. Macroregenerative nodule of the liver: a clinicopathologic study of 345 autopsy cases of chronic liver disease. Cancer. 1988;61:99–105.
31. Wada K, Kondo F, Kondo Y, Large regenerative nodules and dysplastic nodules in cirrhotic livers: a histopathologic study. Hepatology. 1988;8:1684–8.
32. Giorgio A, Francica G, Stefano G, et al. Sonographic recognition of intraparenchymal regenerating nodules using high frequency transducers in patients with cirrhosis. J Ultrasound Med. 1991;10:355–9.
33. Ohtomo K, Itai Y, Ohtomo Y, et al. Regenerating nodules of liver cirrhosis: MR imaging with pathologic correlation. Am J Roentgenol. 1990;154:505–7.
34. Terada T, Nakanuma Y. Iron-negative foci in siderotic macroregenerative nodules in human cirrhotic liver. Arch Pathol Lab Med. 1989;113:916–20.
35. Terada T, Nakanuma Y, Hoso M, et al. Fatty macroregenerative nodule in nonsteatotic liver cirrhosis: a morphologic study. Virchows Arch. 1989;415:131–6.
36. Matsui O, Kadoya M, Kameyama T, et al. Adenomatous hyperplastic nodules in the cirrhotic liver: differentiation from hepatocellular carcinoma with MR imaging. Radiology. 1989;173:123–6.
37. Muramatsu Y, Nawano S, Takayasu K, et al. The diagnosis of small hepatocellular carcinoma: MR imaging. Radiology. 1991;181:209–13.
38. Mano I, Yoshida H, Nakabayashi K et al. Fast spin echo imaging with suspended respiration: gadolinium enhanced MR imaging of liver tumours. J Comput Assist Tomogr. 1987;11:73–80.
39. Schmiedl U, Koelbel G, Hess CF, Kurtz B. Dynamic sequential MR imaging of focal liver lesions using Gd-DTPA: Initial experience in 20 patients. J Comput Assist Tomogr. 1990;4:600–7.
40. Matsui O, Takashima T, Kadoya M, et al. Liver metastases from colorectal cancers: detection with CT during arterial portography. Radiology. 1987;165:65–9.
41. Dodd GD, Miller WJ, Baron RL, Skolnick ML, Campbell WL. Detection of malignant tumors in end-stage cirrhotic livers: efficacy of sonography as a screening technique. Am J Roentgenol. 1992;159:727–33.
42. Miller WJ, Federle MP, Campbell WL. Diagnosis and staging of hepatocellular carcinoma: comparison of CT and sonography in 36 liver transplantation patients. Am J Roentgenol 1991;157:303–6.
43. Chezmar JL, Nelson RC, Malko JA, Bernardino ME. Hepatic iron overload: diagnosis and quantification by noninvasive imaging. Gastrointest Radiol. 1990;15:27–31.
44. Seltzer SE. Janoff AS, Blau M, et al. Biodistribution and imaging characteristics of iotrolan-carrying interdigitation-fusion vesicles. Invest Radiol. 1991;26:S169–71.
45. Miller DL, Rosenbaum RC, Sugarbaker PH, et al. Detection of hepatic metastases: comparison of EOE-13 computed tomography and scintigraphy. Am J Roentgenol. 1983;141:931–5.
46. Schuhmann-Giampieri G, Schmidt-Willich H, Press WR, Negishi C, Weinmann HJ, Speck U, Preclinical evaluation of Gd-EOB-DTPA as a contrast agent in MR imaging of the hepatobiliary system. Radiology. 1992;183:59–64.
47. Hamm B, Vogl TJ, Branding G, et al. Focal liver lesions: MR imaging with Mn-DPDP—initial clinical results in 40 patients. Radiology. 1992;183:53–8.
48. Rofsky NM, Weinreb JC, Bernardino ME, et al. Hepatocellular tumors: characterization with Mn-DPDP enhanced MR imaging. Radiology. 1993;188:53–9.
49. Pavone P, Patrizio P, Buoni C, et al. Comparison of Gd-BOPTA with Gd-DTPA in MR imaging of rat liver. Radiology. 1990;176:61–4.
50. Hoener B-A, Tzika A, Engelstad B, et al. Hepatic transport of the magnetic resonance imaging contrast agent Fe(III)- N-(3-phenylglutaryl) desferrioxamine B. Mag Res Med. 1991; 17:509–15.
51. Fretz CJ, Stark DD, Metz CE, at al. Detection of hepatic metastases: comparison of contrast enhanced CT, unenhanced MR imaging, and iron oxide enhanced MR imaging. Am J Roentgenol. 1990;155:763–70.
52. El Mouaaouy A, Becker HD, Schlief R, Kuhlo C, Portas C. Rat liver model for testing intraoperative echo contrast sonography. Surg Endosc. 1990;4:114–7.
53. Nomura Y, Matsuda Y, Yabuuchi I, et al. Hepatocellular carcinoma in adenomatous hyperplasia: detection with contrast-enhanced US with carbon dioxide microbubbles. Radiology. 1993;187:353–6.
54. Schlief R, Ultrasound contrast agents. Curr Opin Radiol. 1991;3:198–207.
55. Satterfield R, Tarter M, Schumacher J, et al. Comparison of perfluorocarbons as ultrasound contrast agents. Invest Radiol. 1993;28:325–31.
56. Nelson RC, Chezmar JL, Sugarbaker PH, Bernardino ME. Hepatic tumors: comparison of CT during arterial portography, delayed CT, and MR imaging for preoperative evaluation. Radiology. 1989:172:27–34.

# 5

# DETECTION OF LIVER LESIONS: CT-ARTERIAL PORTOGROPHY VS CONTRAST-ENHANCED CT AND MRI

M.E. BERNARDINO

My first experiences with computed angio-portography or computed angio-tomography (CTA or CTAP) of the liver began about sixteen years ago at M.D. Anderson. At the time of its introduction it was a technique that was viewed with a degree of scepticism by clinicians and it has taken a considerable time for it to become more widely accepted, both in the USA and worldwide. Even now, although it is being used much more prior to surgery in patients with hepatocellular carcinoma and colon carcinoma, it is still a highly invasive technique. It is not suitable for use in all cases and so the techniques does have restrictions.

The essence of the technique is the injection of contrast medium via a catheter placed in the hepatic artery, celiac access or the small mesenteric artery (SMA). Originally developed for use in the hepatic artery, the Japanese improved on the technique by placing the catheter in the SMA. Using the SMA is a simpler technique but it must be emphasized that these are two very different techniques with a common denominator; the catheter is placed in an artery, the patient is moved to the CT table, injected with contrast medium and scanned. The computed tomographic angiogram is usually performed with a 5-inch (12.5-cm) catheter placed in the common hepatic artery. Our technique uses 3 ml of contrast medium per second for a total volume of 50–60 ml, with a 6-second delay before scanning. This technique uses the natural physiology of the liver: almost all liver tumours are supplied from the hepatic artery and therefore the tumour has a very dense peripheral blush. With this technique tumours appear white against the normal black hepatic background.

Our technique for portograms is different. Here the catheter is placed either in the SMA or the splenic artery, a much simpler technique. Contrast medium is introduced at the rate of 3 ml per second for a total volume of about 60 ml, with a scan delay of 9–12 seconds. This scan delay is less than that used by most who employ the technique. Digital arteriography shows that the portal vein is normally seen at 9 seconds or less and so the aim is to scan very quickly on the up-slope of the enhancement curve. Because the tumour is not fed from the portal vein it appears as a negative defect in a greatly enhanced liver (Figure 5.1).

There are some interesting features about this technique. It is possible, for example, to evaluate tumour extent – especially in patients with hepatoma. Viewing the portogram, there is a triangular wedge-shaped defect distal to the obstructed portal vein because no iodine is being delivered to that part of the liver. On the arteriogram there is a triangular area of increased enhancement distal to the obstructed portal vein. This is because there are arterial portal anastamoses which open up when the portal vein is obstructed.

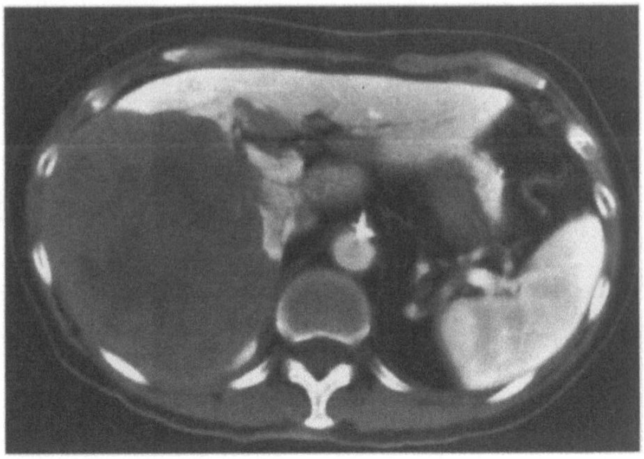

**Figure 5.1** CT portogram demonstrates a large lesion in the right hepatic lobe. Notice that the lesion is a negative defect and the greatly enhanced surrounding normal liver

CT lesion detection rate is about 40–60%, which is equal to MR. Nevertheless even with good quality imaging routinely one half of lesions are missed. CTAP has a detection rate of 85% and if this is analysed further on the basis of the size of lesions, most of the newly detected lesions found by CTAP are less than 1 cm in size. This is significant when considering cancer of the colon as this is the type of patient where there may be recurrence and where these small lesions need to be detected prior to surgery. These smaller lesions are the most difficult to categorize because it is not easy to be tissue-specific about them. So the value that CTAP brings is in detecting lesions smaller than a centimetre in size and it is, currently, the most accurate technique for doing so pre-operatively.

Can another modality help? This is a key question because CTAP by itself still misses between 15 and 20% of lesions in the liver.

Our own work showed that the addition of MR with CTAP gave a 95% lesion detection sensitivity. These data offer some hope and a goal to aim for; that using a contrast agent should be at least equal to the sensitivity of using these two techniques together. Routine imaging has a 50% sensitivity so there is a minimum increase of 25% in sensitivity and it is possible to conceive of an increase of up to 45% in sensitivity with the use of a contrast agent.

A major pitfall of this and most diagnostic techniques is determining the nature of the very small lesions, less than 1 cm in size, that are detected (Figure 5.2). What is a cyst, what is a regenerating nodule, and what is malignant? So the other major goal is tissue specificity.

Our group has looked at more than 1000 CT scans for lesions less than 1 cm in size. In more than 200 we found such masses and it was seen that, in 44–50% of such cases referred with cancer, the lesion was benign. In patients that are non-cancerous and with a lesion of less than 1 cm in size, then 100% of the time it is benign. This is a very interesting finding.

Can we really tell something about this type of lesion? Does it really improve the patient's outcome after surgery?

Before looking at this further, let us consider what the pitfalls of CTAP are. Not only is there the difficulty that we are not sure what these lesions are but the technique also has some real problems such as abnormal catheter placement. In the time that it takes to put the catheter in and move the patient to the CT scanner, the catheter may become displaced. There may be other problems with anatomy, such as replaced right hepatic arteries etc, and with injection rates and contrast density. Also the cardiac output of the patient and the timing of the contrast injection may be a little different. The most common problem, I believe, is really the perfusion defect of 'pseudo-lesions'.

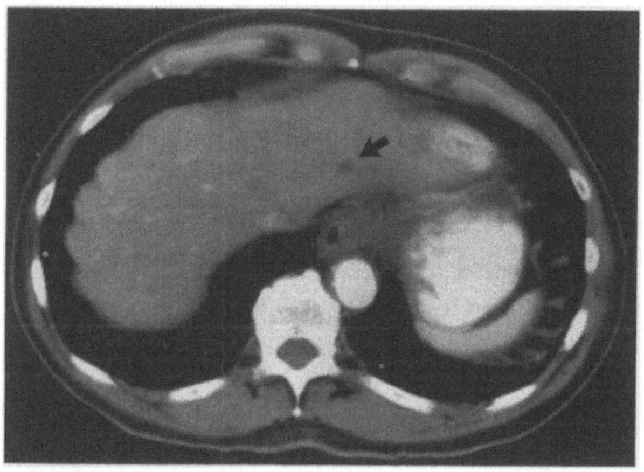

**Figure 5.2** CT section demonstrates a small hypodense lesion in the left hepatic lobe. The lesion is less than 1 cm in size. What is its aetiology? In the non-oncological patient this most likely is benign (cyst/haemangioma). In the cancer patient, less than half of these lesions will be malignant.

If excessive amounts of iodine are used during placement of the catheter in either the SMA or coeliac artery then the sensitivity of the technique is decreased, because iodine moves very rapidly from the intravascular to the extravascular space. Iodine is an extracellular contrast agent and has a tendency to equilibrate in the liver. This is the reason that the NIH paper had a very poor sensitivity to CTAP. They gave 300 ml of 76% contrast before they carried out the CTAP. It is very important that no iodine be used in the placement of the catheter or this results in a poor technique (poor sensitivity for hepatic mass detection).

Other pitfalls of CTAP are due to perfusion defects. One of the most common areas is the posterior medial segment of the left hepatic lobe. Most perfusion techniques are associated with straight lines and are located peripherally in the liver.

Also, in cirrhotic patients, on the arterial side, it is almost impossible for us to identify a focal lesion except when they are very gross. Another type of pseudo-mass is the regenerating nodule. Is it an HCC?

At present we are employing a dual catheter technique. One catheter is placed in the SMA and one in the celiac access. The portogram is done first, and then immediately after this, the arteriogram. By using this technique the number of perfusion defects is decreased.

The importance of any test is whether it really does something that helps people. A recent trial carried out jointly at John Hopkins, Emory, and Washington University–St. Louis involved 404 patients selected for CTAP. The basis of the selection was their possible surgery for either colon carcinoma or hepatocellular carcinoma, although there were also some other tumours present. Tables 5.1 and 5.2 show the number of patients that were deemed to be resectable after CTAP, on the basis that they had, depending upon the surgeon, four or less lesions confined either to one lobe or the liver periphery. So, two-thirds of the patients referred were spared unnecessary surgery and this is a very important point to stress since it means that CTAP does help prior to surgery; it stops two-thirds of patients having unnecessary surgery.

Looking at the data further, in those patients that did have surgery it shows that the technique is not perfect and the accuracy was around 85%. The patients that caused poor sensitivity had metastases that were not hepatocellular carcinoma or colonic

**Table 5.1 CTAP/Surgical database**

| *Primary tumour* | *Total patients* | *Patients determined to be resectable by CTAP* | | *Patients who underwent hepatic resection* | |
|---|---|---|---|---|---|
| Colorectal CA | 197 | 76 | (38.6%) | 69 | (90.8%) |
| Hepatocellular CA | 84 | 39 | (46.4%) | 33 | (84.6%) |
| All others | 123 | 31 | (25.2%) | 20 | (64.5%) |
| Total | 404 | 146 | (36.1%) | 122 | (83.6%) |

**Table 5.2 Accuracy of CTAP in predicting operative findings**

| *Primary tumour* | *CTAP* | *Accuracy* |
|---|---|---|
| Colorectal CA | 69/76 | (90.8%) |
| Hepatocellular CA | 34/39[a] | (87.2%) |
| All others | 21/31[b] | (67.7%) |
| Total | 124/146 | (84.9%) |

[a] Unexpected operative death not included as CTAP error
[b] Patient without liver lesion at surgery and requiring no hepatic resection correctly predicted by CTAP

**Table 5.3 Actuarial yearly survival**

| | *Present study* | *Historical controls* | |
|---|---|---|---|
| | | *Mean* | *Range* |
| 1 year | 88 | 83 | (76–89) |
| 2 year | 77 | 56 | (45–71) |
| 3 year | 66 | 50 | (42–58) |
| 4 year | 51 | 41 | (30–55) |
| <5 year | 24 | | |
| 5 year | | 28 | (22–34) |

carcinoma. What sort of lesions are actually missed by CTAP? We missed, for example, two patients who had very small peripheral, subcapsular metastases that were 1–2 mm in diameter and 1 mm thick. This technique does not pick up such lesions but the majority of lesions that were missed by CTAP were in lymph nodes, both perihepatic and in the coeliac access; these can only be found at surgery. So, this is another limitation of CTAP.

In an extension of the same trial the outcome analysis over a five-year period for all of the patients that went to surgery has been analysed. If these are compared against a historical mean (2000 patients taken from the surgical literature) then the first-year survival rate is roughly the same; the surgery that was performed (even though it is now more aggressive than ten years ago) in these patients did not cause a significant change in outcome.

We are more aggressive now in what we consider is operable. There is, however, a statistical difference in survival at 2, 3 and 4 years if CTAP was performed prior to the resection (Table 5.3). The figures going up to 5 years survival are probably skewed because there were only 8 patients in this group but it is fairly clear that in the first 4 years post-operatively if CTAP is performed prior to colonic section then there is probably at least a 10–15% greater chance, each year, of survival.

Spiral CT has been discussed elsewhere in this volume (Chapter 3). A study at Johns Hopkins comparing 8-mm versus 4-mm CT slices showed that more information was provided when the lesions were 1 cm in size.

Thus, thinner sections provide better data. But, thinner sections are 'noisy'. The advantage of a contrast agent, specifically an hepatic-specific contrast agent, is that it is possible to build the signal and to get much better information. The other feature of spiral CT is that it is possible to obtain volumetric 3D cut-aways. A CT contrast agent changes the situation, making CT more competitive with MR. Spiral CT has extended the use of the modality. The ability to breath-hold liver and cover the entire organ in 15 seconds, with 5-mm sections, has changed our whole approach to this particular organ.

When considering the detection of tumours in the liver, volumes, whether by CT or MR are, I believe, the way that we are going to proceed in the future. Volume imaging, especially as retrospective analysis, requires a contrast agent. The problem with MR in the future is that it operates best at 256 × 256 matrix whereas in CT the equivalent is 512 × 512.

Non-contrast images are noisy and the combination of the use of a contrast agent and changes in technology will become synergistic for sensitivity. Whether they become synergistic for specificity it is not possible to say yet.

Both hepatic-specific MR and CT contrast agents should equal the sensitivity of CTAP and this should be the very minimum goal of a contrast agent. If this goal can be obtained, then both could become the hepatic screening procedures of choice.

## *References*


1. Small WC, Chezmar JL, Bernadino ME. CT angiography and CT arterial portography in evaluation of hepatic adenomas. JCAT 1994;18:266–8.
2. Nelson RC, Thompson GH, Chezmar, JL, Harned RK I, Fernandez MP. CT during arterial portography: diagnostic pitfalls. Radiographics. 1992;12:705–18.
3. Nelson RC. Techniques for computed tomography of the liver. Radiol Clin N Am 1991;29:1199–212.
4. Tyrell RT, Kaufman SL, Bernadino ME. Straight line sign: appearance and significance during CT portography. Radiology. 1989;173:635–7.
5. Nelson RC, Chezmar JL, Sugarbaker PH, Bernadino ME. Hepatic tumours: comparison of CT during arterial portography, delayed CT and MR imaging for preoperative evaluation. Radiology. 1989;172:27–34.
6. Heiken JP, Weyman PJ, Lee JK, Balfe DM, Picus D, Brunt EM, Flye MW. Detection of focal hepatic masses: prospective evaluation with CT, delayed CT, CT during arterial portography and MR imaging. Radiology 1989; 171:47–51.
7. Nelson RC, Chezmar JL, Sugarbaker PH, Murray DR, Bernadino ME. Preoperative localization of focal liver lesions to specific liver segments: utility of CT during arterial portography. Radiology 1990;176: 89–94.

# 6

# SURGICAL ASPECTS IN THE IMAGING OF FOCAL HEPATIC LESIONS

BURCKHARDT RINGE, ARVED WEIMANN
AND RUDOLF PICHLMAYR

## Introduction

The particular surgical interest with regard to focal lesions of the liver is directed towards three main areas which will be discussed subsequently in this article: diagnostic tools, differential diagnosis and indication for surgery; surgical therapy and modalities; patient survival and prognosis. First of all, there are two crucial questions to be asked by the surgeon (Figure 6.1):

1. *Is there any indication at all for surgery*? The answer clearly depends on the aetiology and character of the lesion. As a principle, tumours can be differentiated into benign or malignant types. Fairly common and well-known benign solid tumours are cavernous haemangioma, focal nodular hyperplasia (FNH), and hepatocellular adenoma. While, in haemangioma and FNH, spontaneous rupture and intraperitoneal bleeding are extremely rare, and also malignant transformation is still in discussion in only very few cases of FNH, these particular complications have been reported to occur in adenoma[1–6]. Therefore, it is our own strategy in patients with the clearly established diagnosis of haemangioma or FNH to recommend surgical resection only in cases of symptomatic disease and/or tumour growth. In contrast, due to the risks as described above, surgery for cure should always be performed not only in suspected but also in clearly diagnosed cases of adenoma [2, 4–10]. The question of indication for treatment is somewhat easier in primary or malignant hepatic tumours. Since the spontaneous prognosis is usually fatal within a limited period of time, and currently no alternative effective therapy is available, radical surgery with the aim of potentially curative tumour removal is undoubtedly the treatment of first choice whenever possible.

2. *Is the hepatic lesion resectable*? In order to answer this very important question before operation most precisely, all information available about the anatomy of the lesion must be taken together: exact localization, size and number of the tumours within and outside the liver, as well as involvement of vascular or biliary structures, regional lymph nodes, neighbouring and distant other organs. These data are a prerequisite, not only to decide about the surgical resectability, but also to have an accurate tumour classification and staging which has significant implications for the overall prognosis, especially of patients with malignancies. There are different staging systems in use for primary and also secondary malignant tumours of the hepatobiliary system. At present, most suitable for clinical application seems to be the TNM classification of the International Union against Cancer[11]. Of course, apart from anatomic resectability, the functional capacity of the liver (e.g. in cirrhosis) and the patient's clinical condition must be taken into consideration before surgery.

| Etiology | (Tumor type) | ➡ Indication for treatment |
|---|---|---|

**Benign:** hemangioma, FNH, adenoma, cyst, abscess — or — **Malignant:** primary (HCC, CCC), secondary (CR mets)

| Anatomy | (Tumor stage) | ➡ Surgical resectability |
|---|---|---|

Intrahepatic location, size, number (vascular, biliary structures)
Regional lymph node status
Distant extrahepatic growth

**Figure 6.1** Crucial questions before surgery of focal hepatic lesions. FNH = focal nodular hyperplasia; HCC = hepatocellular carcinoma; CCC = cholangiocellular carcinoma; CR mets = colorectal metastases

## Diagnostic imaging and indication for surgery

In patients with focal hepatic lesions who are referred to a specialized hepatobiliary unit, very often the previous medical history, underlying or accompanying diseases, general clinical status, liver function tests and tumour markers already point in the direction of a typical and specific disease with either a suspected or even a clearly established diagnosis. Thus, the aim of further diagnostic work up is mostly the confirmation of a precise diagnosis with special regard to the questions asked above in the introduction.

At the Medizinische Hochschule, Hannover, we have had a major interest in surgery and transplantation for various hepatobiliary diseases and tumours for many years, and we have always tried to develop specific protocols and strategies for diagnosis and therapy. Thus, in our own hands, the basic different diagnostic tools in use and applied as an interdisciplinary approach by several institutions are the following: sonography as the first examination, which is usually performed by the general practioner outside the hospital, when available in combination with colour Doppler flow analysis; computerized tomography with bolus injection of contrast media; blood pool scintigraphy including SPECT (single photon emission computerized tomography); cholescintigraphy; magnetic resonance imaging; arteriography and indirect mesentericoportography.

Many of the non-invasive investigations can already deliver very tumour-specific results. For example, and focusing on haemangioma and FNH, it is usually possible to diagnose these particular lesions with a high degree of specificity: almost 100% for cholescintigraphy in the identification of FNH, and 98% for blood pool-scintigraphy in the identification of haemangioma[12–14]. The application of invasive procedures for the diagnosis of focal hepatic lesions has become more or less an exception. In our own opinion, which is also confirmed by others, routine fine-needle or core biopsy for further cytological or histological studies should not be performed and thus avoided for two reasons. In general, there is no need: as shown, the diagnosis of haemangioma or FNH can usually be established by non-invasive means; in individual cases also the pathological differentiation between FNH, hepatocellular adenoma and carcinoma may be very difficult; and, even more important, a negative biopsy cannot rule out a malignant tumour[2,15]. On the other hand, there is a considerable risk of bleeding in hypervascularized tumours, and especially of seeding of malignant tumour cells[1,2].

Following our own algorithm, including the principles for indication of surgery as outlined above, the first objective would always be to identify lesions such as haemangioma or FNH (Figure 6.2): if at least two different diagnostic procedures clearly confirm the diagnosis with undoubtedly positive findings typical for one of these two tumour entities, our approach is to follow these patients closely and repeat the appropriate imaging at regular intervals – unless they are symptomatic from a large mass or the lesion is growing in size. Whenever this cannot be accomplished, and thus haemangioma or FNH are excluded, there is a definite indication for operation. Arguments for this approach are that adenoma without intratumoural bleeding has no typical features in diagnostic imaging, and that, in patients without verification of haemangioma or FNH, there is a very high likelihood of either adenoma or any malignant tumour where surgery is indicated anyway[3,16–19].

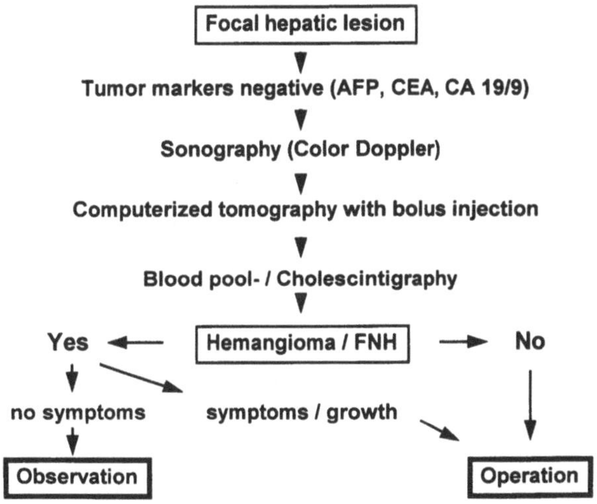


**Figure 6.2** Diagnostic approach and therapeutic consequences for patients with focal hepatic lesions

Of course, liver surgeons are most often consulted by patients with primary or secondary liver cancer as a suspected or already confirmed diagnosis. Hepatocellular carcinoma (HCC) is certainly one of the most common malignancies worldwide with a varying geographical distribution, and a prevalence in Eastern countries and Africa. The association with pre-existing chronic viral hepatitis, and liver cirrhosis is well known. In Europe and North America, probably even more common are liver metastases, especially from primary colorectal cancer. Unfortunately, and despite screening of high-risk groups of patients, many of the malignant tumours found at first presentation are already far advanced with involvement of at least one liver lobe. Whenever technically feasible, anatomic liver resection is the therapy of choice[20–22]. However, in liver cirrhosis, even small tumours may be non-resectable due to functional restrictions. In this particular situation, liver transplantation can be considered as a therapeutic alternative[21–23]. It remains an open issue whether, in potentially resectable early stage I or II hepatocellular carcinoma with underlying cirrhosis, transplantation should be preferred.

## Surgical therapy and techniques

One of the most important prerequisites for modern hepatic surgery is a good knowledge of liver anatomy. From detailed studies and through daily practice, we have learned a lot about the segmental anatomy of the liver parenchyma which is mainly determined by the intrahepatic vascular and biliary architecture[24]. Based on this general experience and the individual lesion to be operated on, various resectional techniques have evolved and can thus be applied. Classical or standard anatomic resections are uni- or plurisegmentectomies, left (including removal of segments I–IV) and right hemihepatectomy (segments V–VIII). Those conventional procedures can be modified and extended with a high degree of flexibility to more or less any type of combination according to the individual tumour and liver anatomy. In principle, dissection and transection of the vascular and biliary structures within the hepatic hilum, and at the level of the hepatic veins is followed by division of the hepatic parenchyma along the anatomic planes. Blood loss can be significantly reduced by an exact anatomical preparation, and meticulous surgical haemostasis, and also by partial inflow occlusion or complete vascular isolation techniques.

In case of more extended resectional procedures the ischaemic tolerance can be improved by additional hypothermic perfusion with specific preservation solutions[25]. Based on the experience from transplantation, the various modifications of in-, ante- or ex-vivo resection as a backtable ('bench') procedure and autotransplantation of the liver have been developed recently[26]. Certainly, the most extensive technique to remove hepatobiliary tumours is total hepatectomy and subsequent liver allotransplantation[21–23]. Radical surgery can be extended even more by multivisceral resection including the liver and other organs, followed by replacement of the liver only or a so-called organ 'cluster'[27]. From the oncological point of view, the true prognostic value of these very advanced procedures remains to be seen in the future. We believe strongly, however, that the present therapeutic strategies of malignant liver tumours should include not only radical surgery but also non-surgical techniques, such as chemoembolization, leading to a multimodality approach on the basis of the individual tumour type and stage[28].

## Patient survival and prognosis after surgery for malignant liver tumours

Despite significant achievements in diagnostic imaging and surgical technique, our common and major interest must be directed towards improving the prognosis of patients, especially those suffering from malignant tumours, and all possibilities available to improve their situation. As an example, hepatocellular carcinoma has an extremely bad spontaneous prognosis with survival in the range of a few months only. On the other hand, it has been clearly shown that partial liver resection can significantly improve this outcome, depending on tumour stage and patient selection. In Asia, resection of small hepatocellular carcinoma was followed by 5-year survival rates of 60–80% again emphasizing the question about epidemiological differences between the eastern and western types of HCC[29].

Our own experience with over 200 patients who had either liver resection or transplantation for hepatocellular carcinoma, shows a 5-year survival rate of about 40% for resection in patients without underlying cirrhosis, and 20% for transplantation (Figure 6.3). Of course, in the transplant group, there were more advanced tumour stages. Looking at survival data, it is very important to know the tumour stages. In accordance with the TNM classification, the survival data for stage II after resection and transplantation show significantly better overall results compared with late stage IV. One has to realize also that patient survival directly depends on the extent of oncological surgery. This means that surgery should always aim at a so-called RO resection – leaving behind no macroscopic or microscopic tumour residues. When looking at the whole population of patients afflicted, in fact, this goal is achieved only in a minority – despite the use of already far-advanced surgical techniques, also emphasizing the need for further improvement of diagnostic

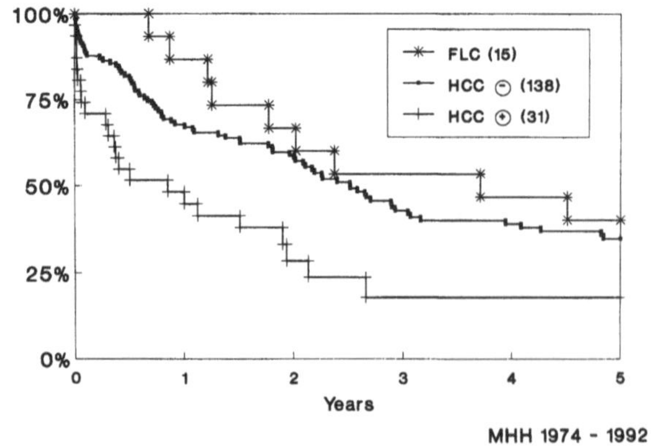


**Figure 6.3** Actuarial patient survival in hepatocellular carcinoma after liver resection. HCC–/+ = hepatocellular carcinoma without/with cirrhosis; FLC = fibrolamellar carcinoma

imaging procedures to detect the tumours at earlier stages and with more accuracy.

Regarding colorectal liver metastases, our own data reveal an overall survival rate for resection in the range of 20–30% after five years which is comparable to the results from other groups (Figure 6.4). In this retrospective analysis, the only significant prognostic factors apart from surgical extent were size, and uni- or bilobar distribution of the lesion[30]. There have been different multicentre studies attempting to determine all relevant prognostic factors. However, many of the factors did not reach statistical significance[31]. Summarizing, it became obvious that a locally limited tumour, unilobar metastases, and absent signs of extrahepatic spread are the most important indicators for less-advanced disease, and thus give a better general prognosis for patients with colorectal metastases. This issue, however, will require even more attention in the future.

The role of liver transplantation as the ultimate approach for otherwise non-resectable hepatic lesions due to anatomical or functional restrictions has stimulated a lot of controversial but still ongoing discussions, despite disappointing general results worldwide[21–23,32–37]. This may, in part, be related to the acceleration of tumour growth and recurrence due to the influence of immunosuppression[38]. With special regard to the overall shortage of donor organs, there is almost general agreement that primary liver tumours, like advanced hepatocellular carcinoma stage IV, cholangiocellular carcinoma, and haemangiosarcoma, have to be considered contraindications for liver transplantation[39]. More uncommon tumour entities, like the fibrolamellar carcinoma, epithelioid haemangioendothelioma or hepatoblastoma, seem to have a more favourable long-term outcome (Figure 6.5). In the case of secondary liver malignancies, the results are extremely bad for colorectal metastases, but significantly better for metastases from neuroendocrine tumours (Figure 6.6). Split-liver transplantation may be an alternative to overcome the limited donor resources, at least temporarily. Using an appropriate dissection technique, the left part of the liver can be transplanted fairly safely in the same way as the already established standard procedure of partial liver transplantation to a small child, usually with a benign disease, while the right part, with more risk from necessary reconstruction of the vascular structures, can be made available to an adult patient with a

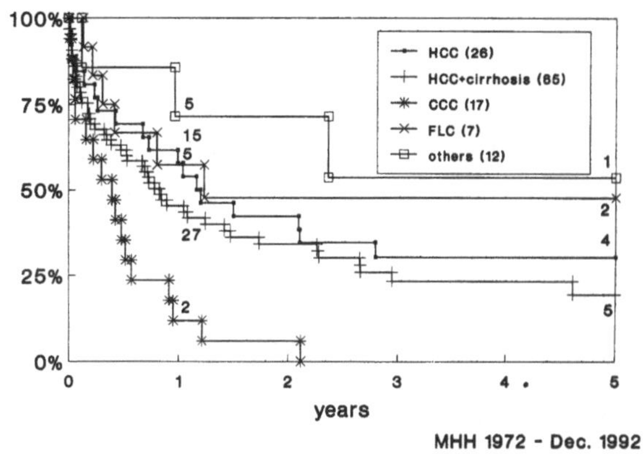


**Figure 6.5** Actuarial patient survival in different entities of primary hepatic tumour after liver transplantation. HCC = hepatocellular carcinoma; CCC = cholangiocellular carcinoma; FLC = fibrolamellar carcinoma

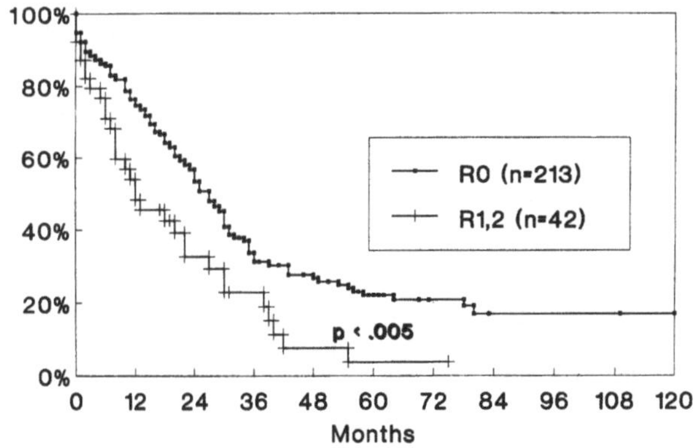


**Figure 6.4** Actuarial patient survival in colorectal liver metastases after hepatic resection. R0 = no residual tumour; R1,2 = microscopic/macroscopic residual tumour

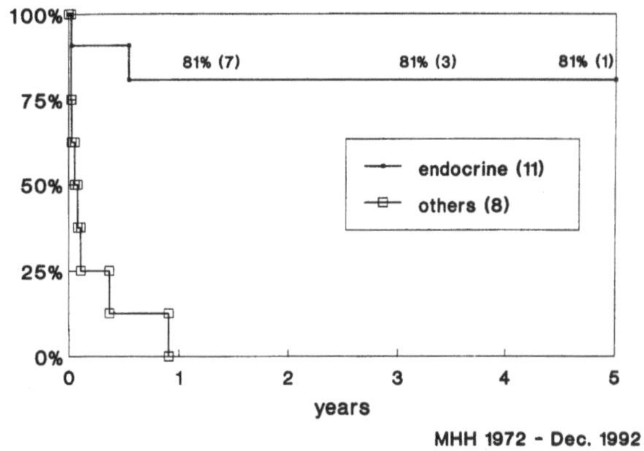


**Figure 6.6** Actuarial patient survival in secondary liver tumours after hepatic transplantation according to aetiology

malignant tumour who might otherwise have no chance of a donor organ in time[40].

## Summary and conclusions

For patients with focal hepatic lesions, non-invasive procedures should be preferred in the diagnostic work-up. By combination of different imaging procedures, haemangioma and FNH can be diagnosed with a high degree of specifity and safety – followed by close observation of the lesion, while surgery has only to be discussed in cases with tumour-related symptoms and/or growth. In contrast, for all other tumours and without clear verification of their diagnosis, there is an absolute indication for surgery. This also includes adenoma, with the potential risk of tumour rupture, and especially malignant transformation. In primary and secondary hepatobiliary malignancy, exact tumour staging by preoperative diagnostic work-up remains the basis and gold standard to decide about appropriate treatment modalities, and to identify and select those patients who will benefit most from surgery. Most of the present staging systems rely on at least one piece of information which can only be obtained by operative exploration or histopathological examination of a surgically taken specimen. This is of special relevance for vascular tumour infiltration and extrahepatic lymph node status. Here, further improvement can be expected by future development of less-invasive techniques, e.g. by the use of laparoscopic sonography.

In conclusion, an accurate diagnosis and adequate therapy are the most essential prerequisites, both contributing to improvement in the prognosis for patients with focal hepatic lesions. As Martin Adson, certainly one of the pioneers in modern liver surgery, stated some years ago: ‘We clearly have the need for better imaging techniques not only to cure the patient but also our own blindness to each tumour's real stage’[41].

### *References*


1. Hobbs KEF. Hepatic hemangiomas. World J Surg. 1980; 14:468–71.
2. Iwatsuki S, Todo S, Starzl TE. Excisional therapy for benign hepatic lesions. Surg Gynecol Obstet. 1990;171: 240–6.
3. Kerlin P, Davis GL, McGill DB, Weiland LH, Adson MA, Sheedy PF. Hepatic adenoma and focal nodular hyperplasia: clinical, pathologic and radiologic features. Gastroenterology. 1983;84:994–1002.
4. Leese T, Farges O, Bismuth H. Liver cell adenomas. A 12-year experience from a specialist hepato-biliary unit. Ann Surg. 1988;208:558–64.
5. Nichols FC, van Heerden JA, Weiland LH. Benign liver tumors. Surg Clin N Am. 1988;69:297–314.
6. Trastek VF, van Heerden JA, Sheedy II PF, Adson MA. Cavernous hemangiomas of the liver: Resect or observe? Am J Surg. 1983;145:49–53.
7. Foster JH. Benign liver tumors. World J. Surg. 1982; 6:25–31.
8. Lise M, Feltrin G, Da Pian PP, Miotto D, Pilatti PL, Rubaltelli L, Zane D. Giant cavernous hemangiomas: diagnosis and surgical strategies. World J Surg. 1992;16:516–20.
9. Ringe B, Mauz S, Barg-Hock H, Kotzerke J. Pichlmayr R. Chirurgie bei beningnen Lebertumoren. Langenbecks Arch Chir Suppl II. 1989;(Kongreßbericht 1989):287–91.
10. Weil III, Koep LJ, Starzl TE, Liver resection for hepatic adenoma. Arch Surg. 1979;114:178–80.
11. Hermanek P, Sobin LH, eds. TNM classification of malignant tumors. 4th fully revised ed. Berlin: Springer; 1987:56–9.
12. Gratz KF, Creutzig H, Brölsch C, Neuhaus P, Majewski A, Pichlmayr R, Hundeshagen H. Choleszintigraphie zum Nachweis der focal-nodulären Hyperplasie (FNH) der Leber? Chirurg. 1984;55:448–51.
13. Kotzerke J, Schwarzrock R, Krischek, Wiese H, Hundeshagen H. Technetium 99m DISIDA hepatobiliary agent in diagnosis of hepatocellular carcinoma, adenoma and focal nodular hyperplasia. J. Nucl Med. 1989;30:1278–9.
14. Kudo M, Ikekubo K, Yamamoto K, Ibuki Y, Hino M, Tomita S, Komon H, Orino A, Todo A. Distinction between haemangioma of the liver and hepatocellular carcinoma: value of labeled RBC-SPECT scanning. Am J Roentgenol. 1989; 152:977–83.
15. Müller-Leisse C, Kujat Ch, Klose K, Büchsel R. Diagnostik der Fokal nodulären Hyperplasie. Röntgenpraxis. 1990;43:281–7.
16. Ros PR, Li KCP. Part II: Benign liver tumors. Curr Probl Diagn Radiol. 1989;May/June:125–55.
17. Sandler MA, Petrocelli RD, Marks S, Lopez R. Ultrasonic features and radionuclide correlation in liver cell adenoma and focal nodular hyperplasia. Radiology. 1980;135:393–7.
18. Welch TJ, Sheedy PF, Johnson CM, Stephens DH, Charboneau JW, Brown ML, Ray GR, Adson MA, McGill DB. Focal nodular hyperplasia and hepatic adenoma: comparison of angiography, CT, US and scintigraphy. Radiology. 1985;156:593–5.
19. Weimann A, Barg-Hock H, Klempnauer J, Gratz KF, Grote R, Kotzerke J, Lang H, Wagner S, Ringe B, Pichlmayr R. Wertigkeit der Sonographie bei der Diagnostik und Verlaufskontrolle von Hämangiom und Fokal Nodulärer Hyperplasie der Leber. Ultraschall Klin Prax. 1994;[in press].
20. Gozzetti G, Mazziotti A, Grazi GL, Jovine E, Gallucci A, Morganti M, Frena A, Agucro V, Cavallari A. Surgical experience with 168 primary liver cell carcinomas treated by hepatic resection. J. Surg Oncol (Suppl). 1993;3:59–61.
21. Iwatsuki S, Starzl TE, Sheahan DG, Yokoyama I, Demetris AJ, Todo S, Tzakis AG, Van Thiel DH, Carr B, Selby R, Madariaga J. Hepatic resection versus transplantation for hepatocellular carcinoma. Ann Surg. 1991;214:221–9.
22. Ringe B, Pichlmayr R, Wittekind C, Tusch G. Surgical treatment of hepatocellular carcinoma: Experience with liver resection and transplantation in 198 patients. World J Surg. 1991;15:270–85.
23. Bismuth H, Chicle L, Adam R, Castaing G. Surgical treatment of hepatocellular carcinoma in cirrhosis: Liver resection or transplantation? Transplant Proc. 1993;25:1066–7.

24. Couinaud C. Surgical anatomy of the liver revisited. Paris: Depot legal:2ieme trimestre: 1989.
25. Fortner JG, Shiu MH, Kinne DW, Castro EB, Watson RC, Howland WS, Beattie EJ. Major hepatic reactions using vascular isolation and hypothermic perfusion. Ann Surg. 1974;180:644–52.
26. Pichlmayr R, Grosse H, Hauss J, Gubernatis G, Lamesh P, Bretschneider HJ. Technique and preliminary results of extracorporeal liver surgery (bench procedure) and of surgery on the in situ perfused liver. Br J Surg. 1990; 77:21–6.
27. Starzl TE, Todo S, Tzakis A, Podesta L, Mieles L, Demetris A, Teperman L, Selby R, Stevenson W, Stieber A, Gordon R, Iwatsuki S. Abdominal organ cluster transplantation for the treatment of upper abdominal malignancies. Ann Surg. 1989; 210:374–85.
28. Galanski M, Schmoll E, Reichelt S, Böhmer G, Prokop M, Schaefer C, Schüler A, Ringe B, Schmidt FW, Schmoll HJ. Chemoembolisation hepatozellulärer Karzinome bei isoliertem Leberbefall. Radiologe. 1992;32:49–55.
29. Tang ZY, Yu YQ, Zhou XD, Yang BH, Ma ZC, Lin ZY. Subclinical hepatocellular carcinoma: An analysis of 391 patients . J Surg Oncol (Suppl). 1993;3:55–8.
30. Ringe B, Bechstein WO, Raab R, Meyer HJ, Pichlmayr R. Leberresektion bei 157 Patienten mit colorektalen Metastasen. Chirurg. 1990;61:272–9.
31. Scheele J, Stang R, Altendorf–Hofmann A, Gall FP. Indicators of prognosis after hepatic resection for colorectal secondaries. Surgery. 1992;110:13–29.
32. O'Grady JG, Polson RJ, Rolles K, Calne RY, Williams R. Liver transplantation for malignant disease. Results in 93 consecutive patients. Ann Surg. 1988;207:373–9.
33. Ringe B, Wittekind C, Bechstein WO, Bunzendahl H, Pichlmayr R. The role of liver transplantation in malignancy. A retrospective analysis with special regard to tumour stage and recurrence. Ann Surg. 1989;209:88–98.
34. Ismail T, Angrisani L, Gunson BK, Hübscher SG, Buckels JAC, Neuberger JM, Elias E, McMaster P. Primary hepatic malignancy: The role of liver transplantation. Br J Surg. 1990;77:983–7.
35. Olthoff K, Millis M, Rososve MH, Goldstein LI, Ramming KP, Busuttil RW. Is liver transplantation justified for the treatment of hepatic malignancies? Arch Surg. 1990;125:1261–8.
36. Haug CE, Jenkins RL, Rohrer RJ, Auchincloss H, Delmonico FL, Freeman RB, Lewis WD, Cosimi AB. Liver transplantation for primary hepatic cancer. Transplantation. 1992; 53:376–82.
37. Moreno-Gonzalez EM, Gomez R, Garcia I, Gonzalez-Pinto I, Loinaz C, Ibanez J, Bercedo J, Palomo JC, Palma F, Vorwald P, Riano D, Perez Cerda F, Davila P, Cisneros C, Maffettone V, Sciadini M. Liver transplantation in malignant hepatic neoplasms. Am J Surg. 1992;163:395–400.
38. Yokoyama I, Carr B, Saitsu H, Iwatsuki S, Starzl TE. Accelerated growth rates of recurrent hepatocellular carcinoma after liver transplantation. Cancer. 1991;68:2095–100.
39. Pichlmayr R, Weimann A, Ringe B. Indications for liver transplantation in hepatobiliary malignancy. Hepatology. 1994, [in press].
40. Pichlmayr R, Ringe B, Gubernatis G, Hauss J, Bunzendahl H. Transplantation einer Spenderleber auf zwei Empfänger (Splitting-Transplantation) – Eine neue Methode in der Weiterentwicklung der Lebersegmenttransplantation. Langenbecks Arch Chir. 1988;373:127–30.
41. Adson MA. Editorial comment. Am J Surg. 1987;156:372.

# 7

# POTENTIALS OF NEW MRI CONTRAST AGENTS IN THE CHARACTERIZATION OF LIVER MALIGNANCIES

G. MARCHAL AND Y. NI

## Introduction

The differential diagnosis of focal liver lesions by plain magnetic resonance imaging (unenhanced MRI) is based on different parameters: (1) morphological appearance in T1 and T2 sequences; and (2) quantitative criteria such as signal intensity T1 and T2 values. The combination of these parameters has obviously improved the differentiation of the main types of focal liver lesions (metastases, haemangioma, cysts, HCC and focal–nodular hyperplasia etc.). Nevertheless, the value of this differential diagnosis remains limited because of overlap in the MRI findings of benign and malignant liver tumours. Because of these limitations, the need for additional parameters has been rapidly recognized. Today, non-specific gadolinium-based chelates are routinely used to assess lesion vascularization. Unfortunately, because of the rapid extravascular diffusion of regular gadolinium-chelates, their potential in the liver is limited to dynamic studies after a short bolus injection, similar to contrast-enhanced (CE) CT. Though the diagnostic accuracy of current MRI of the liver already surpasses that of CE CT, a number of new liver-specific agents is currently under development, in the hope of further improving the diagnostic value of MRI, both in terms of detection and characterization.

*Liver-specific contrast agents (CA)* can be categorized into two large groups: (1) particulates, such as the small and ultrasmall particles of iron oxide, liposomes etc., which target either the Kupffer cells or the hepatocytes; (2) ionic agents, such as manganese dipyridoxal diphospate (Mn-DPDP), and gadolinium-ethoxybenzyl (Gd-EOB-DTPA), which are metabolized by the hepatocytes. *Tumour-specific CA*, a new category currently under investigation, are designed to be taken up exclusively by tumour cells. Metalloporphyrins may yield this expectation.

Most of the preclinical and clinical studies with these components have been designed to assess the improvement in lesion *detection*[1–3]. Until now, relatively little attention has been paid to their value for improved lesion *characterization.* However, a reliable differentiation of focal liver lesions is crucial for adequate diagnostic and therapeutic decisions.

We report from our experience on the value of Mn-DPDP, Gd-EOB-DTPA, metalloporphyrins, and iron oxide particles for liver tumour characterization. The data shown were obtained in preclinical studies with well-defined animal models of primary and secondary liver tumours.

## Mn-DPDP

The new MR contrast agent, manganese dipyridoxal diphosphate (Mn-DPDP) is a manganese chelate derived from pyridoxal 5′-phosphate. It has been biochemically designed to be secreted by the hepatocyte into the bile. In rats and rabbits, peak relaxation enhancement of liver tissue occurs at approximately 30 minutes after injection. It is slowly cleared by the liver with a 50% decrease in the maximal enhancement approximately 2 hours after injection[4–6].

As a liver-specific contrast agent, Mn-DPDP has been used to improve the conspicuity of focal liver lesions. Promising results were first shown in laboratory animals with implanted liver tumours[7]. More recently, this experimental finding has been confirmed by the multicentre phase II clinical trials in patients with liver metastasis and hepatocellular carcinoma (HCC)[8–10]. In patients with liver metastases, the improved visualization after injection of Mn-DPDP is due to the strong liver enhancement which occurs almost immediately after administration and lasts for at least 6 hours. Liver metastases showed only a minimal enhancement so that the overall liver–lesion contrast-to-noise ratio (CNR) was improved, i.e. negative enhancement. They also observed varying degrees of Mn-DPDP uptake by HCC lesions, i.e. positive enhancement.

In order to obtain a better insight into different mechanisms of primary liver cancer enhancement by Mn-DPDP, an animal study was set up in which the enhanced MR images of HCCs were correlated with their corresponding histology. Primary liver cancer was chemically induced in rats[11]. Microangiography and Gd-DOTA were used to evaluate the accessibility of the contrast media to each individual HCC lesion and to assess the non-specific contribution of Mn-DPDP to tumour enhancement.

Light microscopy was used to evaluate the influence of cellular differentiation and relative tumour cell volume on specific tumour enhancement.

Mn-DPDP is actively taken up and metabolized by differentiated primary hepatocellular tumours. Contrast uptake is multifactorial and depends on tumour differentiation, accessibility and cell quantity. The enhancement caused by selective intracellular uptake is further non-specifically increased by the intravascular fraction of Mn-DPDP during the early phase after injection. Animal studies demonstrated that only differentiated HCCs showed a positive Mn-DPDP enhancement persisting for more than 48 hours (Figure

7.1a,b). In these lesions, the highest conspicuity score appeared 24 hours after the injection. However, all undifferentiated HCCs were delineated by a prompt negative enhancement with maximal conspicuity within 30 minutes. This observation suggest that both early (within the first hour) and delayed (at 24 hours) scans are equally important for better detection and characterization of liver tumours. This aspect should be considered in the design of future clinical studies[12].

In addition during both animal and clinical MRI studies, positively enhancing rims around liver tumours have been observed[12,13]. In order to elucidate the origins of these rims and to assess their potential value in the differential diagnosis, a total of 69 primary and secondary liver cancers were studied (14). Mn-DPDP and Gd-DOTA enhanced MR images were compared. On the Mn-DPDP enhanced images, 34 peritumoural rims of various patterns were observed. All of them occurred in highly malignant primary and secondary liver tumours (Figure 7.2a–c). Comparison between the MR images with the corresponding microangiography and histology showed that these rims are related to peritumoural zones of malignant infiltration, surrounding parenchyma compression and bile duct proliferation[14].

## Gd-EOB-DPTA

Gadolinium-ethoxybenzyl-DTPA (Gd-EOB-DTPA) is characterized by a high affinity to the hepatocytes and an important biliary excretion. Gd-EOB-DTPA enters the hepatocyte via a specific carrier-mediated protein and is subsequently excreted in the biliary plexus[15,16]. As Mn-DPDP, it was also designed to cause positive enhancement of the liver parenchyma, leaving the hepatic tumours as *negative defects*. The efficacy of Gd-EOB-DTPA in this regard has been

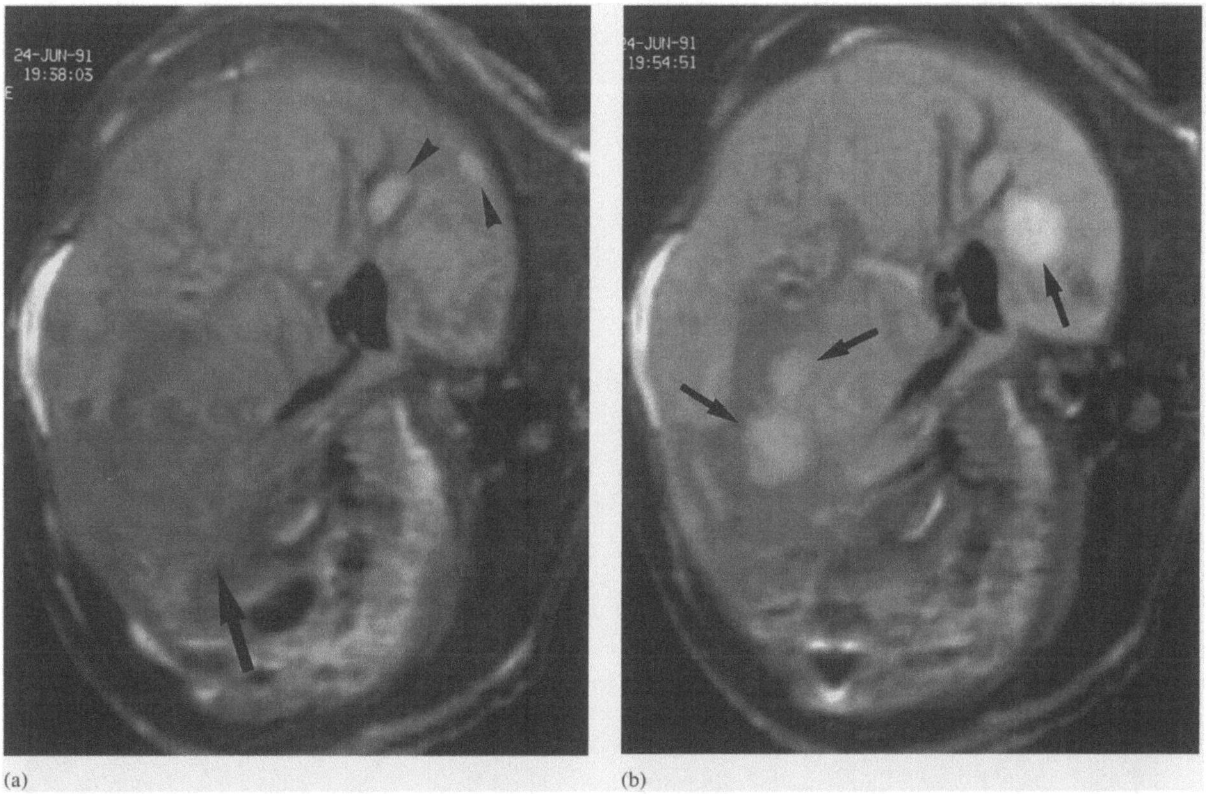


(a) (b)

**Figure 7.1** Chemically induced hepatocellular carcinoma in the rat. a. Precontrast T1-weighted (TR/TE: 600/15 ms) spin echo (T1W SE) image. Inhomogeneous hypointense area in the left lobe (thick arrow) is due to extensive cirrhotic changes. Only two small slightly hyperintense lesions in the posterior aspect of the right liver lobe are visible (arrowheads). b. Ten minutes after the injection of Mn-DPDP (25 $\mu$mol/kg, Byk Gulden, Konstanz, Germany), three additional positively enhancing lesions can be detected (arrows). Notice the different degree of uptake, mainly related to differences in cellular differentiation on histology. This positive enhancement persists for more than 48 hours, with highest conspicuity at 24 hours due to normalization of the liver intensity

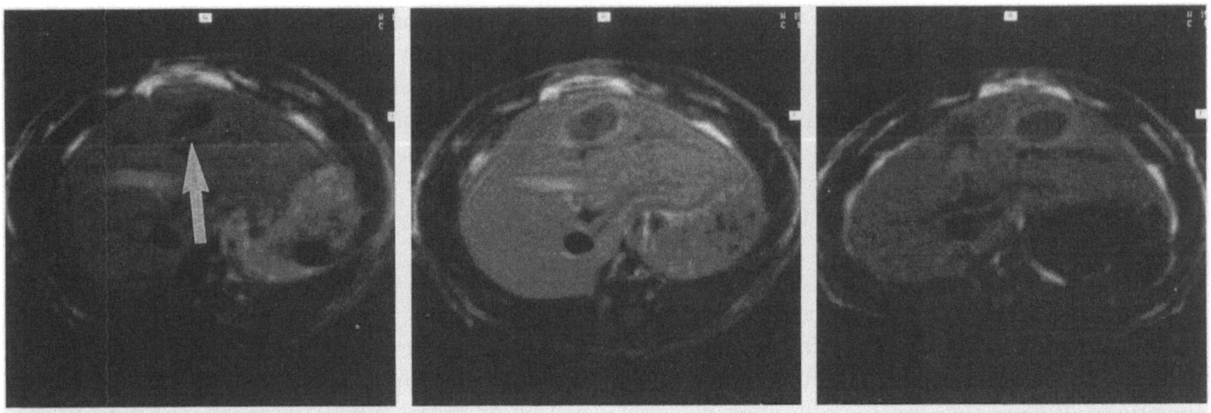

(a) (b) (c)

**Figure 7.2** Implanted Novikoff hepatoma in the rat. a. Precontrast T1W SE image. The tumour is seen as a hypointense nodule with a faint hyperintense rim (arrow). b. Ten minutes after Mn-DPDP injection, the liver is intensely enhanced and the tumour now becomes better delineated with a strongly enhanced peripheral rim. c. 24 hours after Mn-DPDP injection, with the signal intensity of the liver returning to the precontrast level, the rim sign is even more conspicuous due to delayed elimination of the agent from the peritumoural liver parenchyma. Corresponding histology showed scattered tumour infiltration in this peritumoural region

demonstrated in models of implanted liver tumour[3,17]. A similar finding in primary liver cancer was also shown in a comparative study with Mn-DPDP[18].

In contrast to Mn-DPDP, Gd-EOB-DTPA shows negative enhancement in almost all primary liver cancers (Figure 7.3a,b), with the only exception in highly differentiated HCCs, showing prolonged positive enhancement (Figure 7.4a–d). This finding implies that uptake of Gd-EOB-DTPA relies on a higher level of hepatocytic function. It might be helpful in discriminating highly differentiated hepatocyte-derived benign and malignant tumours from other liver malignancies.

Though less pronounced than with Mn-DPDP, enhancing rims are also seen around undifferentiated or implanted liver tumours after Gd-EOB-DTPA

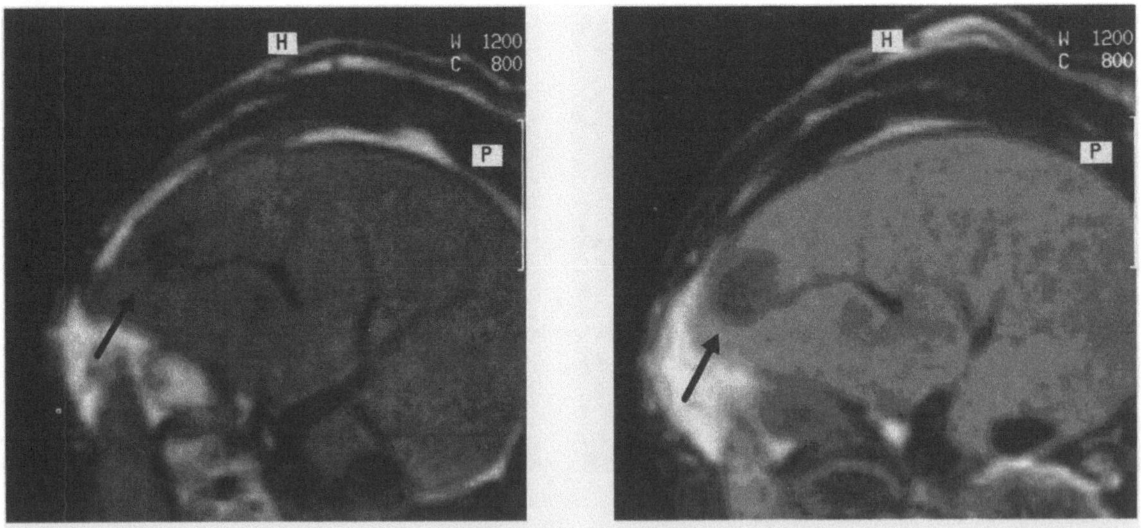


(a) (b)

**Figure 7.3** Chemically induced hepatocellular carcinoma in the rat. a. Precontrast T1W SE image. The arrow points to a tumour that appears hypointense. b. Ten minutes after the injection of Gd-EOB-DTPA (30 $\mu$mol/kg, Schering, Berlin, Germany), an improved conspicuity of the liver tumour (arrow) is obtained due to a negatively increased tumour–liver contrast to noise ratio (negative enhancement). The histology of the tumour corresponds to an undifferentiated HCC

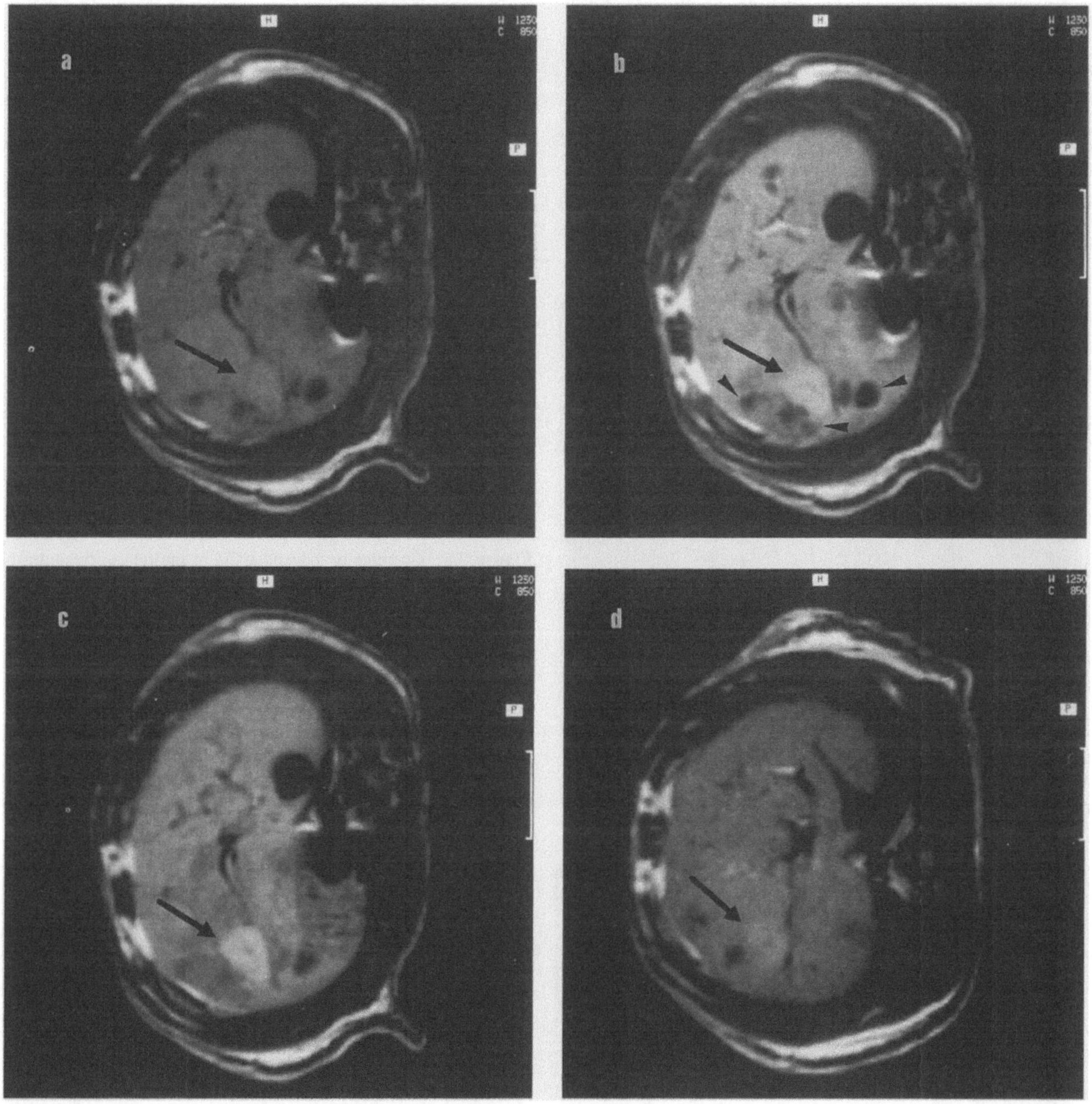


**Figure 7.4** Chemically induced hepatocellular carcinoma in the rat. a. Precontrast T1W SE image. The arrow points to a solid, almost isointense, nodule surrounded by a number of small hypointense lesions. b. Ten minutes after the injection of Gd-EOB-DTPA, the liver parenchyma becomes diffusely enhanced. Pronounced positive enhancement of the large nodule (arrow) is shown, in contrast with the non-enhancing surrounding nodules (arrowheads). c. 30 minutes after Gd-EOB-DTPA injection, the large nodule (arrow) shows the highest conspicuity, accompanied by a rapid decay of the liver enhancement. d. At 24 hours' follow-up, the Gd-EOB-DTPA is completely eliminated from the large nodule (arrow), as well as from the liver parenchyma. Notice that the duration of the positive tumour enhancement induced by Gd-EOB-DTPA is much shorter than that by Mn-DPDP (approximately 2 hours versus 48 hours). The histology of this Gd-EOB-DTPA positively enhanced nodule indicates a highly differentiated HCC

injection. Here also, malignant infiltration into the surrounding parenchyma seems to be the principal cause of this phenomenon.

### Metalloporphyrins

The potential of the tumour-specificity of two metalloporphyrins, Gd-haematoporphyrin (Gd-HP) and Mn-tetraphenylporphyrin (Mn-TTP), has recently been studied in the same comprehensive models of liver tumours. At the early phase after administration, both metalloporphyrins behaved similarly to the non-specific Gd-DTPA and enhanced tumours by perfusion and diffusion. However, delayed images after 24–48 hours showed moderate contrast retention in certain compartments of some tumours. Histology of these areas revealed intratumoural necrosis, thrombosis or secretions (Figure 7.5a–c). Similar uptake was also seen in inflammatory

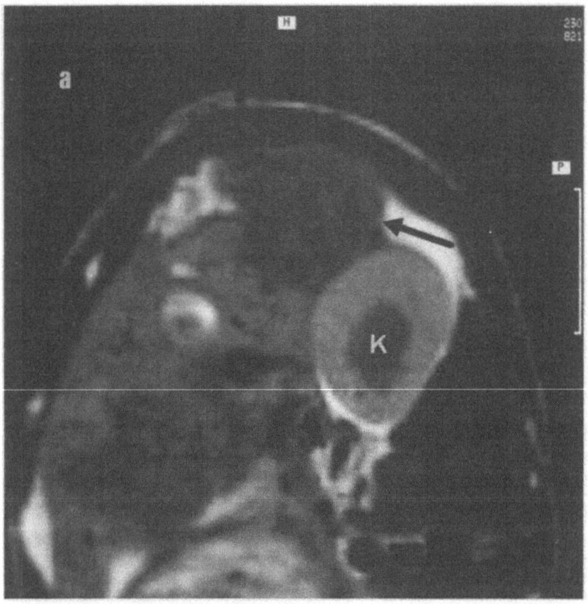


**Figure 7.5** Chemically induced HCC in the rat. a. Precontrast T1W SE image reveals a hypointense tumour located at the lower edge of the right liver lobe (arrow). K indicates the right kidney. b. Ten minutes after the injection of Mn-TPP (50 $\mu$mol/kg, IDF, Berlin, Germany), strong enhancement of the peripheral part of the tumour (arrow) can be seen, without enhancement of the central area. c. At 24 hours' follow-up after Mn-TPP injection, a reversed contrast of the central and peripheral parts appears in the tumour (arrow), suggesting a delayed accumulation and retention of the agent within the central part. Histology reveals an extremely vascularized undifferentiated HCC with massive central thrombosis and necrosis corresponding to the delayed central enhancement

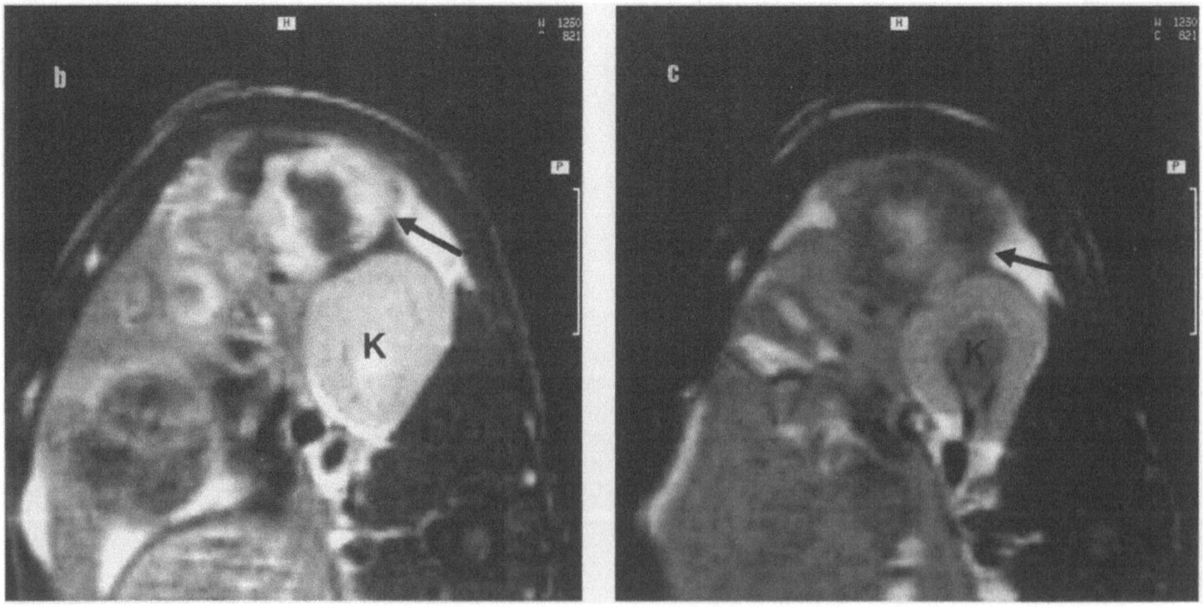

lesions. Therefore, the agents studied cannot be regarded as specific for viable tumour cells. This finding is different from some studies on similar hydrophilic metalloporphyrins[19–25] but in agreement with the results of other investigators[26,27].

As suggested by recent papers[28–30], a possible explanation for this failure of tumour specifity is that the porphyrins used in this study are more hydrophilic than the porphyrins used in cancer photodynamic therapy. The latter are highly lipophilic and can therefore preferentially enter the tumour cells by addressing the LDL receptors which are particularly abundant on tumour cell membranes.

## RES-specific contrast agents

Iron oxide-based RES (reticuloendothelial system)-specific contrast media have been most extensively studied in preclinical studies and have already entered clinical trials.

Once injected, these particulate agents are rapidly cleared from the blood by the monocytic macrophage system (or RES) of the body. In this regard, the Kupffer cells in the liver play a dominant role. Increased liver lesion conspicuity is based on the absence of Kupffer cells in almost all space-occupying lesions, with, as the only exception, the benign hepatocyte-derived solid lesions. The iron oxides, stored in the Kupffer cells, induce strong local susceptibility effects that destroy the liver signal on moderately T2 weighted SE or gradient echo images, leaving the focal liver lesions as bright spots[31,32].

Contrast uptake in a tumour indicates the presence of active Kupffer cells and can therefore be used to identify focal nodular hyperplasia and adenoma. However, absence of uptake does not exclude a benign primary tumour, nor does scattered uptake exclude the possibility of a highly differentiated hepatocellular carcinoma (Figure 7.6a,b).

## Conclusion

The relatively high sensitivity of MRI to MR contrast agents allows the development of substances with pharmacokinetic behaviour similar to that of hepatobiliary scintigraphic agents used in nuclear medicine.

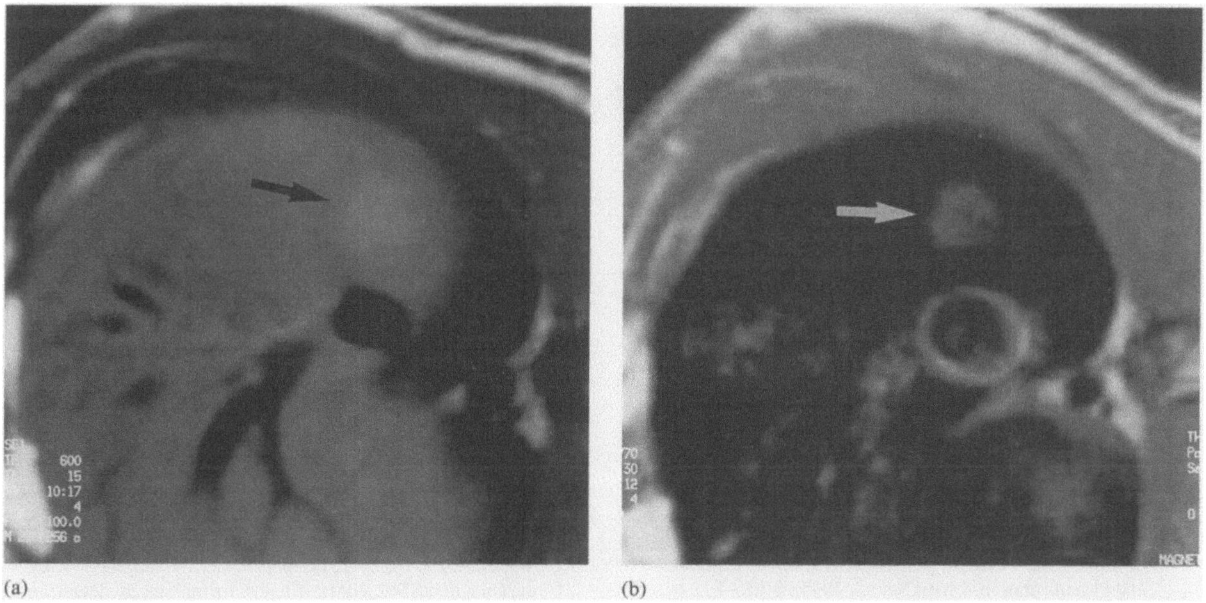

**Figure 7.6** Chemically induced HCC in the rat. a. Precontrast T1W (TR/TE: 600/15 ms) SE image. A slightly hyperintense lesion (arrow) on the right liver lobe can be seen. b. Moderately T2W (TR/TE: 770/30 ms) SE image. 20 minutes after the injection of carboxydextran-coated iron oxide particles (30 $\mu$mol/kg, Schering, Berlin, Germany), the lesion (arrow) stands out positively due to drastic blackening of the normal liver parenchyma. Notice some scattered iron oxide uptake inside the lesion, suggesting some phagocytosis of the particle by the remaining RES within the tumour. Histology of the tumour revealed a well-differentiated HCC

Though the doses that have to be injected are relatively large, relevant signal changes can be obtained without risk to the patients.

CE MRI has an advantage over nuclear medicine, by offering besides functional information, improved anatomical resolution. One can therefore expect that many of the new molecules currently under investigation will not only increase lesion detection but also improve non-invasive lesion characterization.

## *References*


1. Stark DD, Elizondo G, Fretz CJ. Liver-specific contrast agents for MRI. Invest Radiol. 1990;25:S58.
2. Saini S. Contrast-enhanced MR imaging of the liver. Radiology. 1992;182:12–14.
3. Clement O, Mühler A, Vexler VS, Kuwatsuru R, Berthezene Y, Rosenau W, Brash RC. Comparison of Gd-EOB-DTPA and Gd-DTPA for contrast-enhanced MR imaging of liver tumours. J Magn Reson Imaging. 1993;3:71–7.
4. Rocklage SM, Caaheris WP, Quay SC, Hahn FE, Raymond KN. Manganese (II) N, N′-dipyridoxylethylenediamine-N, N′-diacetate 5,5′-bis (phosphate): synthesis and charazterization of a paramagnetic chelate for magnetic resonance imaging enhancement. Inorg Chem. 1989;28:477–85.
5. Elizondo G, Fretz CJ, Stark DD, et al. Preclinical evaluation of MnDPDP: new paramagnetic hepatobiliary contrast agent for MR imaging. Radiology. 1991;178:73–8.
6. Nelson RC, Chezmar JL, Newberry LB, et al. Manganese dispyridoxyl diphosphate: effect of dose, time, and pulse sequence on hepatic enhancement in rats. Invest Radiol. 1991;26:569–73.
7. Young SW, Bradley B, Muller HH, Rubin DL. Detection of hepatic malignancies using Mn-DPDP (manganese dipyridoxal diphosphate) hepatobiliary MRI contrast agent. Magn Reson Imaging. 1990;8:267–76.
8. Rummeny E, Ehrenheim Ch, Gehl HB, et al. Manganese-DPDP as a hepatobiliary contrast agent in the magnetic resonance imaging of liver tumours: results of clinical phase II trials in Germany including 141 patients. Invest Radiol. 1991;26:S142–5.
9. Hamm B, Vogl TJ, Branding G, et al. Focal liver lesions: MR imaging with Mn-DPDP - initial clinical results in 40 patients. Radiology. 1992;182:167–74.
10. Rofsky NM, Weinreb JC, Bernardino ME, Young SW, Lee J, Noz M. Hepatocellular tumours: Characterization with Mn-DPDP-enhanced MR imaging. Radiology. 1993;188:53–9.
11. Ni Y, Marchal G, Van Damme B, Van Hecke P, Michiels J, Zhang X, Yu J, Baert AL. MR imaging, microangiography and histology in a rat model of primary liver cancer. Invest Radiol. 1992;27:689–97.
12. Ni Y, Marchal G, Zhang X, Van Hecke P, Michiels J, Yu J, Rummeny E, Lodemann K-P, Baert AL. The uptake of Mn-DPDP by chemically induced HCC in rats: A correlation between contrast media enhanced MRI, tumor differentiation and vascularization. Invest Radiol. 1993;28:520–8.
13. Rummeny E, Wiesmann W, Menker S, Lodemann K, Peter PE. Value of delayed Mn-DPDP enhanced MR imaging in the detection and differential diagnosis of hepato tumours. J Magn Reson Imaging 1992;2:65.
14. Ni Y, Marchal G, Yu J, Rummeny E, Zhang X, Lodemann K, Baert AL. Experimental liver cancers: Mn-DPDP-enhanced rims in MR-microangiographic-histologic correlation study. Radiology. 1993;188:45–51.
15. Weinmann H-J, Schuhmann-Giampieri G, Schmitt-Willich H, Vogler H, Frenzel T, Gries H. A new lipophilic gadolinium chelate as a tissue-specific contrast medium for MRI. Magn Res Med. 1991;22:233–7.
16. Schuhmann-Giampieri G, Schmitt-Willich H, Negishi C, Weinmann H-J. Preclinical evaluation of Gd-EOB-DTPA as a contrast agent in MR imaging of the hepatobiliary system. Radiology. 1992;183:59–64.
17. Muhler A, Clement O, Vexler V, Berthezene Y, Rosenau W, Brasch RC. Hepatobiliary enhancement with Gd-EOB-DTPA: Comparison of spin-echo and STIR imaging for detection of experimental liver metastases. Radiology. 1992;184:207–13.
18. Marchal G, Zhang X, Ni Y, Yu J, Baert A. Comparison between Gd-DTPA, Gd-EOB-DTPA and Mn-DPDP in induced HCC in rats. A correlation study of MR imaging, microangiography and histology. Magn Reson Imaging. 1993:11(5):14.
19. Chen CW, Cohen J, Myers C, Sohn M. Paramagnetic metalloporphyrins as potential contrast agents in NMR imaging. FEBS Lett. 1984;168:70–4.
20. Patronas N, Cohen J, Knop R, Dwyer A, Colcher D, Lundy J, Mornex F, Hambright P, Sohn M, Myers C. Metalloporphyrin contrast agents for magnetic imaging of human tumours in mice. Cancer Treat Rep. 1986;70:391–5.
21. Lyon R, Faustino P, Cohen J, Katz A. Tissue distribution and stability of metalloporphyrin MRI contrast agents. Magn Reson Med. 1987;4:24–33.
22. Koenig S, Brown III R, Spiller M. The anomalous relativity of $Mn^{3+}$ ($TPPS_4$). Magn Reson Med. 1987;4:252–60.
23. Ogan M, Revel D, Brasch R. Metalloprphyrin contrast enhancement of tumours in magnetic resonance imaging. A study of human carcinoma, lymphoma, and fibrosarcoma in mice. Invest Radiol. 1987;22:822–8.
24. Place D, Faustino P, van Zijl P, Chesnick A, Cohen J. Metalloporphyrins as contrast agents for tumours in magnetic resonance imaging. Invest Radiol. 1990;25:S69–S70.
25. Place D, Faustino P, Berghmans K, van Zijl P, Chesnick A, Cohen J. MRI contrast-dose relationship of manganese (III) tetra (4-sulfonatophenyl) porphyrin with human xenograft tumours in nude mice at 2.0 T. Magn Reson Imaging. 1992;10:919–28.
26. Nelson J, Schmiedl U, Shankland E, SMRM, New York City, Book of Abstracts. 1990;vol 1:232.
27. Nelson J, Schmiedl U. Porphyrins as contrast media. Magn Reson Med. 1991;22:366–71.
28. Kreimer-Birnbaum M. Modified porphyrins, chlorins, phthalocyanines and purpurins: Second-generation photosensitizers for photodynamic therapy. Semin Hematol. 1989;26:157–73.
29. Nelson J, Schmiedl U. Shankland E, Metalloporphyrins as tumor-seeking MRI contrast media and as potential selective treatment sensitizers. Invest Radiol. 1990;25:S71–3.
30. Pass H. Photodynamic therapy in oncology: Mechanisms and clinical use. J Natl Cancer Inst.1993;85:443–56.
31. Saini S, Stark D, Hahn P, Bousquet J-C, Introcasso J, Wittenberg J, Brady T, Ferrucci J. Ferrite particles: A superparamagnetic MR contrast agent for enhanced detection of liver carcinoma. Radiology. 1987;162:217–22.
32. Tsang YM, Stark D, Chen M, Weissleder R, Wittenberg J, Ferruci J. Hepatic micrometastases in the rat: Ferrite-enhanced MR imaging. Radiology. 1988;167:21–4.

8

# FOCAL LIVER LESIONS: MAGNETIC RESONANCE IMAGING–PATHOLOGICAL CORRELATION

PABLO R. ROS

Magnetic resonance (MR) imaging is becoming the non-invasive imaging technique of choice for the liver. This is due to the recent development of what has been called 'advanced MR'. Advanced MR imaging includes modern techniques such as gradient-echo imaging, fast spin echo imaging and fat suppression, as well as MR contrast agents that improve lesion conspicuity and provide physiological information[1,2].

These improvements not only allow an increase in lesion detection but also offer the potential for tissue characterization[3]. In order to be able to characterize focal liver lesions, it is essential to understand their underlying pathological nature.

Gadopentetate dimeglumine or gadolinium-DTPA (Gd-DTPA) is the primary intravenous paramagnetic contrast agent available for general use in MR imaging. Gd-DPTA produces T1 shortening, therefore, appearing bright on T1 weighted (T1W) imaging[4]. Although Gd-DTPA is a vascular agent, it is quickly distributed to the extracellular compartment in both normal liver and focal masses, requiring the use of fast dynamic techniques, such as T1W gradient-echo imaging, to detect differences between normal liver and focal lesions.

At an experimental level in the USA, specific reticuloendothelial system (RES) contrasts are being tested that have the potential to replace functional radionuclide liver imaging, as they produce physiological as well as anatomical information[5,6]. Superparamagnetic iron oxide (SPIO) is a particular agent producing predominantly T2 shortening, and therefore causing decreased signal intensity in all pulsing sequences, especially in T2 weighted (T2W) imaging[5]. SPIO is phagocytosed by RES cells in the liver (Kupffer cells), and is therefore taken up by normal liver, fatty liver and benign tumours composed of hepatocytes.

In this chapter, we review the key microscopic and gross features of the most common benign and malignant liver neoplasms, correlating them with MR imaging findings. Therefore, a pathological–MR imaging 'translation' is offered for each of the neoplasms reviewed[1].

We discuss the most common primary hepatic neoplasms in the adult, both benign (haemangioma, focal nodular hyperplasia and hepatocellular adenoma) and malignant (hepatocellular carcinoma, fibrolamellar carcinoma, intrahepatic cholangiocarcinoma and cystadenoma/cystadenocarcinoma). We are not presenting metastases due to the variable histological and gross appearance, depending upon the primary tumour, nor focal inflammatory lesions (abscesses and echinococcal cysts).

For each neoplasm discussed, a table summarizing the MR and pathological findings is included.

## Haemangioma

### *Pathology*

Haemangioma is the most common hepatic mass, being found in up to 20% of the population. It occurs primarily in women (5:1 ratio compared with men) of any age, although it is frequently discovered during the premenopausal years. Most haemangiomas are clinically silent, becoming symptomatic only when they are large or compressing adjacent structures[7].

Microscopically, haemangiomas are formed by multiple vascular channels, lined with a single layer of endothelial cells supported by a fibrous stroma (Figure 8.1). Very slow blood flow through the lesion is characteristic, leading to areas of thrombosis, hyalination, and eventually fibrosis within the tumour. Calcifications (in the form of phleboliths) are occasionally present.

Grossly, haemangiomas are usually solitary and small (typically less than 4 cm in diameter). Areas of fibrosis are usually present. The tumours are very well delimited, although they do not have a capsule. There are large feeding vessels in the periphery of the tumour (Figure 8.1a). By convention, when a haemangioma is larger than 10 cm, it is called a 'giant haemangioma' and often contains central cleft-like areas of fibrosis (Figure 8.1b)[1].

### *MR imaging*

By MR imaging, haemangioma is a well-marginated mass, usually homogeneous in signal, although potentially heterogeneous, due to areas of thrombosis, fibrosis or haemorrhage[8,9].

On T1W imaging, they have decreased signal intensity relative to normal liver[8,10] (Figure 8.2a). On T2W imaging, haemangiomas are markedly hyperintense with increase of relative signal intensity with increasing echo time (TE) (Figures 8.2b and c). This appearance is due to the slow blood flow through the vascular channels. Areas of fibrosis produce decreased

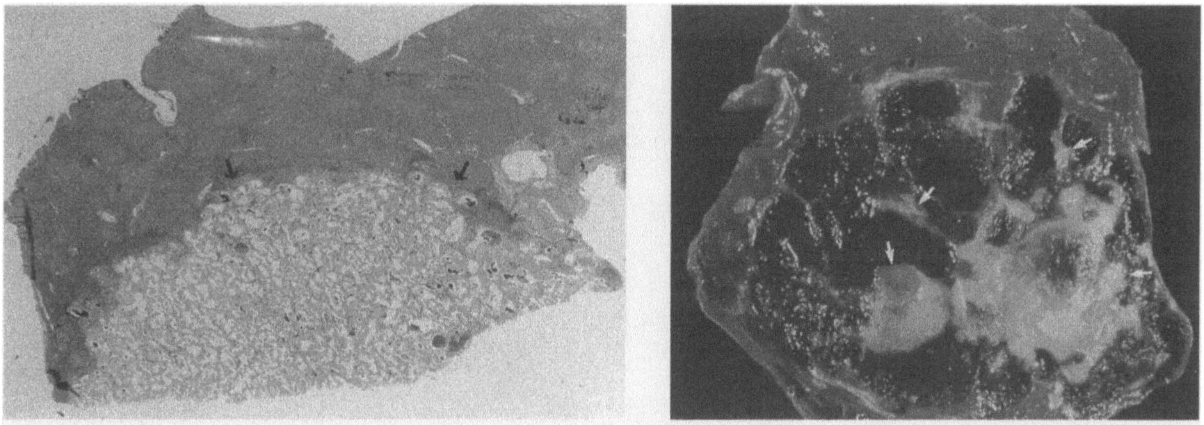

(a) (b)

**Figure 8.1** Hemangioma. **a.** This subgross H&E specimen demonstrates prominent feeding vessels (arrows) and the lesion's well-defined and lobulated margin with the surrounding normal liver. **b.** Fibrotic nodules and bands (arrows) are surrounded by the spongy well-defined tumour in this gross specimen. Areas of haemorrhage and necrosis are also present.

signal intensity, while cystic or haemorrhagic areas are of increased signal intensity[9,11] (Figures 8.2b and 8.2c). Fat-suppressed images demonstrate nicely the sharp margins (Figure 8.2d).

Dynamic gradient-echo images following intravenous (iv) Gd-DTPA (0.05 mmol/kg) typically show peripheral contrast enhancement with subsequent fill-in occurring within 15 minutes (Figures 8.2e, f and g). There is no enhancement in the areas of fibrosis (Figure 8.2h). The prolonged enhancement is due to the characteristic lack of intratumoural shunting[4,12] (Table 8.1).

**Table 8.1 Haemangioma: MRI–pathological correlation**

| *Pathology features* | *MRI appearance* |
|---|---|
| • Well-defined lesion, usually peripheral | • Sharply defined, may be lobulated |
| • Typically solitary, small homogeneous lesion | • Hypointense T1W imaging |
| • Very slow blood flow through vascular channels | • Markedly hyperintense relative to liver on long TE T2W imaging |
| • Fibrosis occasionally | • Areas of decreased signal T2W imaging |
| • Cystic change and haemorrhage | • Areas of increased signal T2W imaging |
| • Giant haemangioma, larger than 10 cm diameter, often contains central fibrosis | • Heterogeneous lesion which may incompletely enhance post-Gd-DTPA |
| • Peripheral feeding vessels | • Centripetal, prolonged enhancement with Gd-DTPA |

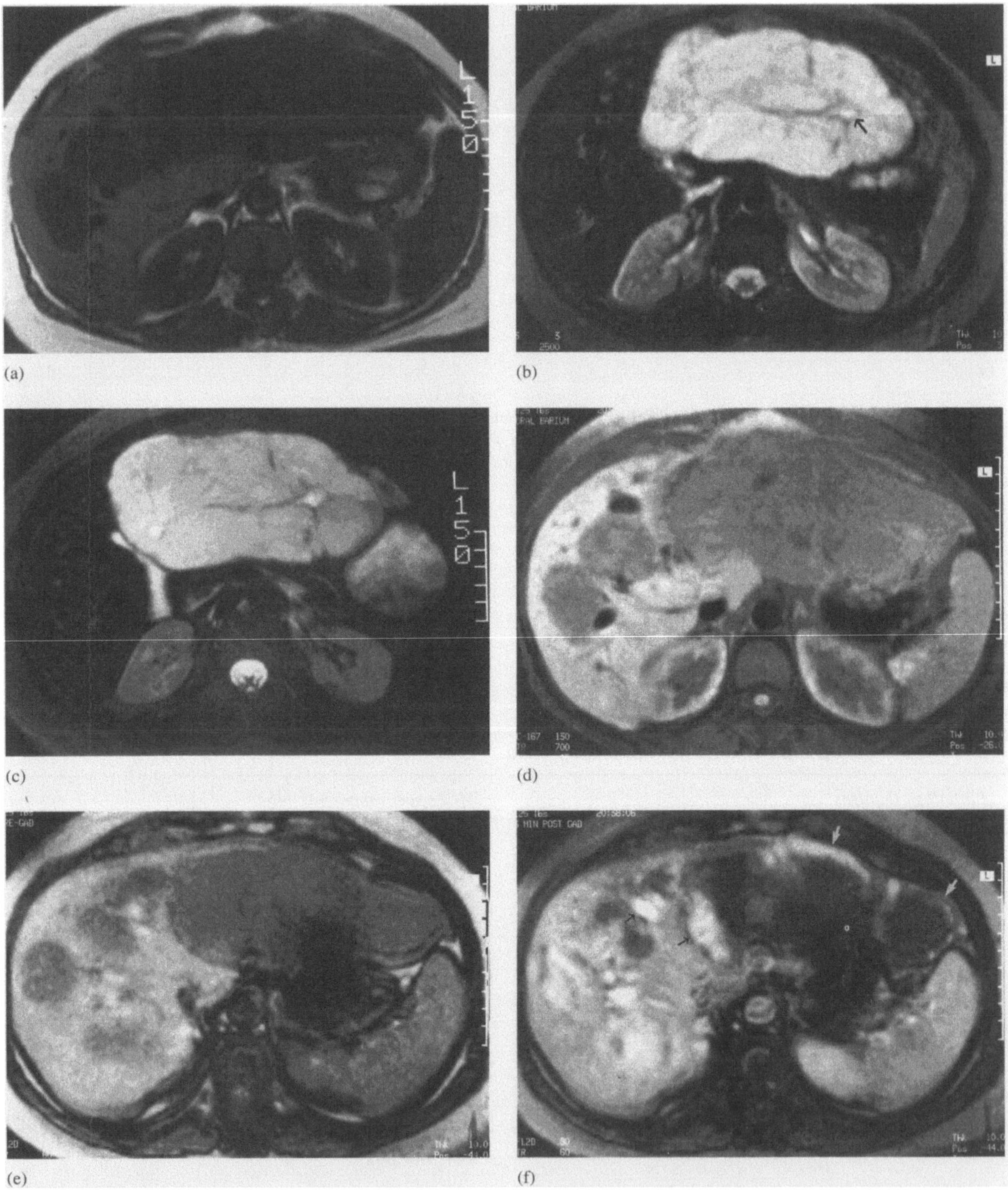

(a) (b) (c) (d) (e) (f)

**Figure 8.2** Giant haemangioma in a 43-year-old woman with upper abdominal pain. **a**. T1W imaging (TR 300/TE 12) demonstrates a large hypointense mass involving the left hepatic lobe and two smaller hypointense lesions within the right hepatic lobe. **b**. T2W imaging (TR 2500/TE 120) through the centre of the large left lobe lesion shows it to be markedly hyperintense. A central scar is present. A focus of higher signal intensity is due to cystic change (arrow). **c**. Fast spin-echo T2W imaging (TR 5500/TE 119) shows better resolution allowing visualization of additional internal scars and cystic areas compared with conventional spin-echo. **d**. Fat-suppression T1W imaging (TR 700/TE 15) reveals the haemangiomas to be of decreased signal intensity relative to normal liver. **e.** Gradient-echo T1W imaging (TR 60/TE 12, 80°) also demonstrates haemangiomas as hypointense. Note lack of high flow vessels within the haemangiomas. **f**. Gradient-echo T1W imaging (TR 60/TE 12, 80°) obtained 3 minutes after iv Gd-DTPA shows peripheral enhancement of the large haemangiomas (arrows) and almost complete filling of the smaller ones.

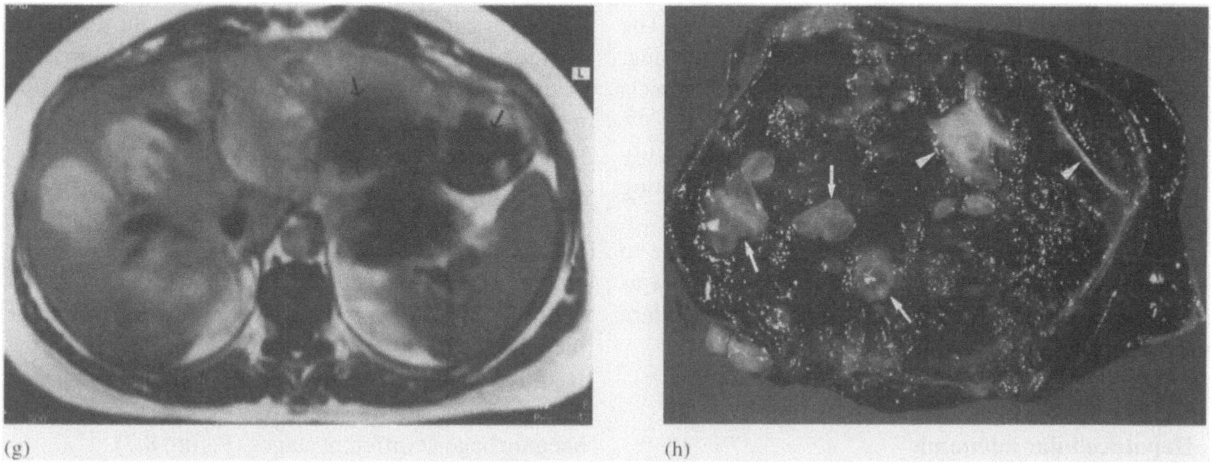

**Figure 8.2** **g**. T1W imaging (TR 300/TE 15) obtained 15 minutes after iv Gd-DTPA demonstrates complete enhancement of the smaller lesions. The central portions of the large mass have not enhanced (arrows). This is often seen in giant haemangiomas due to fibrosis. **h**. In the gross specimen, there are multiple areas of cystic change (arrows). Fibrosis is also present (arrowheads), corresponding with MR imaging findings

## Focal nodular hyperplasia

### *Pathology*

Focal nodular hyperplasia (FNH) is a benign tumour-like condition that is like a hyperplastic response to an underlying congenital arteriovenous malformation[13]. More commonly seen in women, it is usually discovered incidentally in the third to fifth decades of life.

Histologically, a central fibrous scar containing the remnants of the arteriovenous malformation is surrounded by nodules of benign hyperplastic hepatocytes (Figure 8.3a). Although vessels are prominent throughout the lesion, they are most abundant in the scar[14]. The scar does not contain calcifications.

Grossly, FNH is almost always solitary and measures less than 5 cm. On cut section, it is relatively homogeneous, without areas of haemorrhage or necrosis except for the central fibrous scar (Figure 8.3b). Although it has sharp margins, it has no capsule.

### *MR imaging*

On T1W imaging, FNH is isointense, occasionally hypointense, to normal liver[8,14] (Figure 8.4a). On T2W imaging, it is usually isointense to normal liver

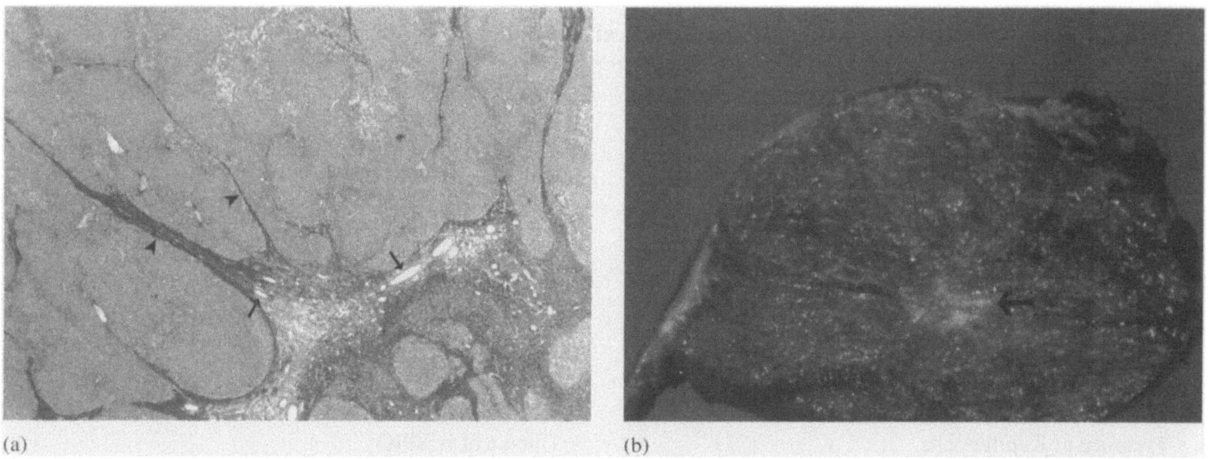

**Figure 8.3** Focal nodular hyperplasia (FNH). **a**. This low-power Masson-stain photograph, in which collagen stains blue, reveals the central scar containing vessels (arrows). Note the multiple radiating septae (arrowheads), creating the typical nodular pattern of FNH. **b**. On cut section, FNH is homogeneous except for central fibrous scar (arrow). (Corresponds to case illustrated in Figure 8.4.)

but occasionally hyperintense (Figure 8.4b)[15,16]. The central scar is usually hyperintense on T2W imaging, despite being fibrous tissue, due to the internal vessels with high-speed flow and oedema (Figure 8.4b)[15,16]. Fat-suppressed T1W imaging depicts the scar richly as a markedly hypointense central area with radiating fibrous strands (Figure 8.4c).

Marked enhancement after iv Gd-DTPA is due to excellent vascularity[17]. SPIO uptake is expected as the lesion contains Kupffer cells and has an excellent vascular supply (Figures 8.4d and e; Table 8.2).

## Hepatocellular adenoma

*Pathology*

The majority of hepatocellular adenomas (HCA) are seen in women of childbearing age who are using oral contraceptives. It is almost never seen in men unless taking anabolic steroids. HCA may rupture and cause haemoperitoneum which leads to this benign tumour being considered as a surgical lesion[18].

Histologically, HCA is comprised of benign hepatocytes which are arranged in sheets and cords, mimicking normal liver architecture. HCA contains Kupffer cells and frequently its hepatocytes are rich in fat and glycogen[19] (Figure 8.5a). However, the lesion lacks portal tracts, hepatic veins, and biliary canaliculi.

Grossly, HCA is typically larger than FNH (5–10 cm at presentation) and frequently surrounded by a fibrous capsule which contains large vessels (Figure 8.5a). On cut section, it has a yellow colour due to fat contents (Figure 8.5a) and often contains areas of haemorrhage or infarction (Figure 8.7b). Pedunculation may be seen in 10% of cases.

*MR imaging*

HCA cannot be distinguished from hepatocellular carcinoma by unenhanced MR imaging (Figures 8.6 and 8.7). On T1W imaging, HCA may contain areas of increased signal intensity relative to normal liver due to fatty change or haemorrhage[20] (Figures 8.6a and 8.7a). Haemosiderin rings can be seen, suggesting haemorrhage at different stages (Figure 8.7).

On T2W imaging, it may demonstrate a heterogeneous appearance with areas of hypeintensity due to central necrosis or haemorrhage[8,21] or be homogeneously slightly hyperintense if necrosis is present (Figure 8.6c). If there is a capsule, it appears as a hypointense rim with large subcapsular feeding vessels. Although the use of RES contrast material has not been reported in HCA, our experience with iv SPIO in a single case showed poor uptake, similar to that in sulphur colloid scans (Figure 8.9; Table 8.3).

## Hepatocellular carcinoma

*Pathology*

Hepatocellular carcinoma (HCC) is the most common primary epithelial neoplasm of the liver[7]. Its incidence and aetiology vary dramatically around the world. In the Western hemisphere, underlying cirrho-

**Table 8.2 Focal nodular hyperplasia: MRI–pathological correlation**

| *Pathology features* | *MRI appearance* |
|---|---|
| • Benign tumour-like condition containing nodules of benign hepatocytes and bile ductules | • Variable appearance on T1W and T2W imaging, often isointense to liver |
| • Central fibrous scar containing a congenital AV malformation | • May have central scar which is hyperintense on T2W imaging |
| • Excellent vascularity | • Marked, prompt enhancement post-iv Gd-DTPA |
| • Presence of Kupffer cells | • Uptake of iv SPIO |

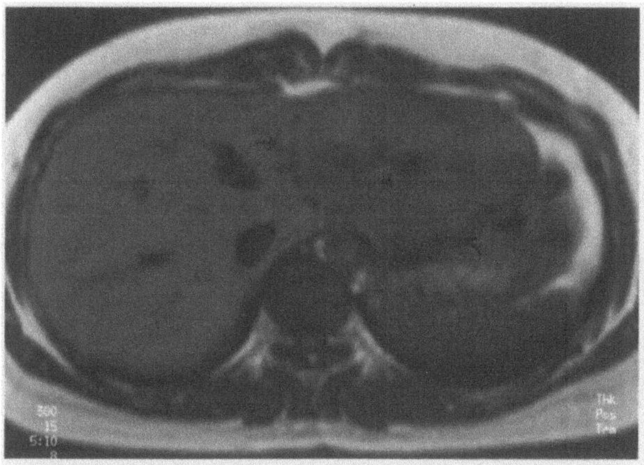

(a)

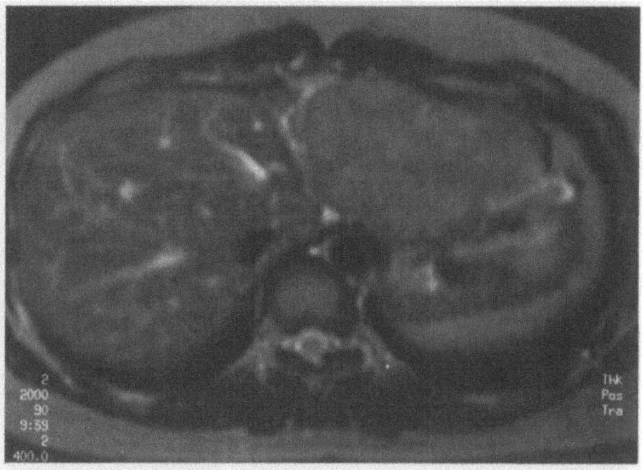

(b)

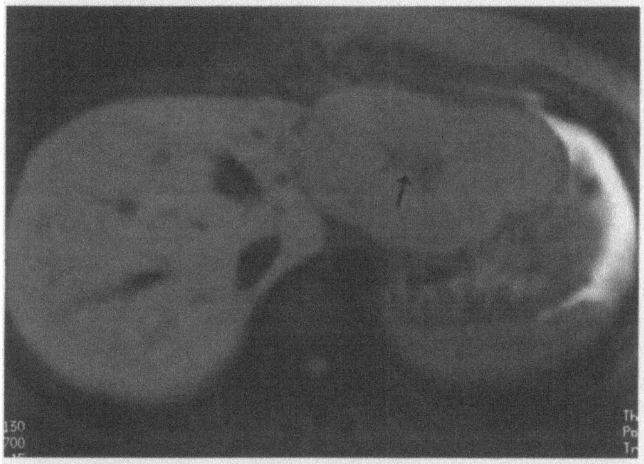

(c)

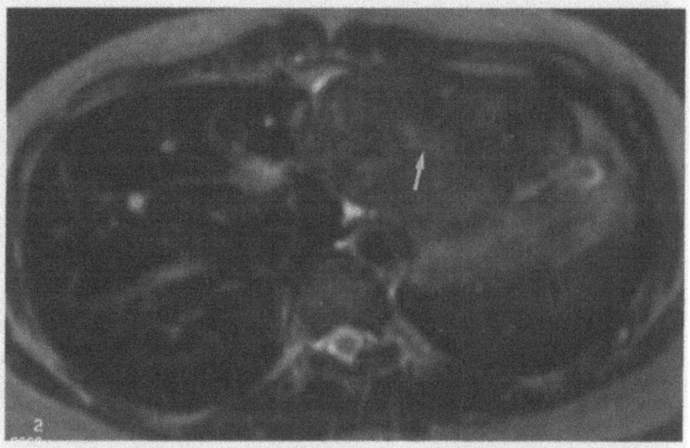

(d)

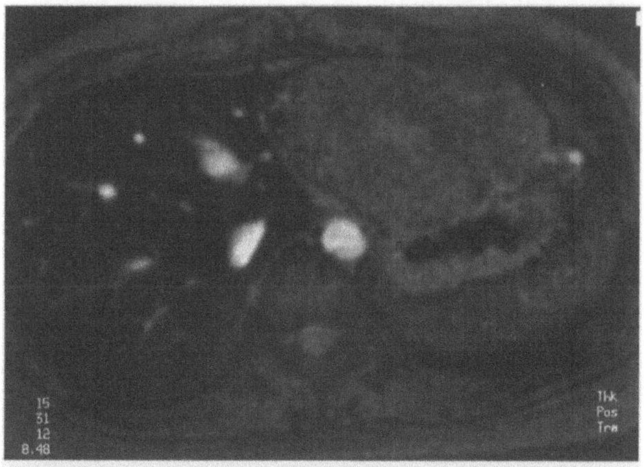

(e)

**Figure 8.4** Focal nodular hyperplasia in a 38-year-old woman. **a**. T1W imaging (TR 300/TE 15) shows a slightly hypointense mass (straight arrows) replacing the lateral segment of the left lobe with a central scar (arrowhead). **b**. T2W imaging (TR 2000/TE 90) reveals the mass to be slightly hyperintense relative to liver. The scar remains hypointense. **c**. Fat-suppression T1W imaging (TR 700/TE 15) shows the lesion to be slightly hypointense. The central scar with radiating septa (arrow) is well displayed. **d**. T2W imaging (TR 2000/TE 90) after iv SPIO shows decrease in signal of both liver and mass, but the scar (arrow) without SPIO uptake remains slightly hyperintense. **e**. Gradient-echo T2W imaging (TR 31/TE 12, 15°) post-iv SPIO accentuates the slight uptake differential between the mass and the liver, further decreasing the relative signal intensity of the liver

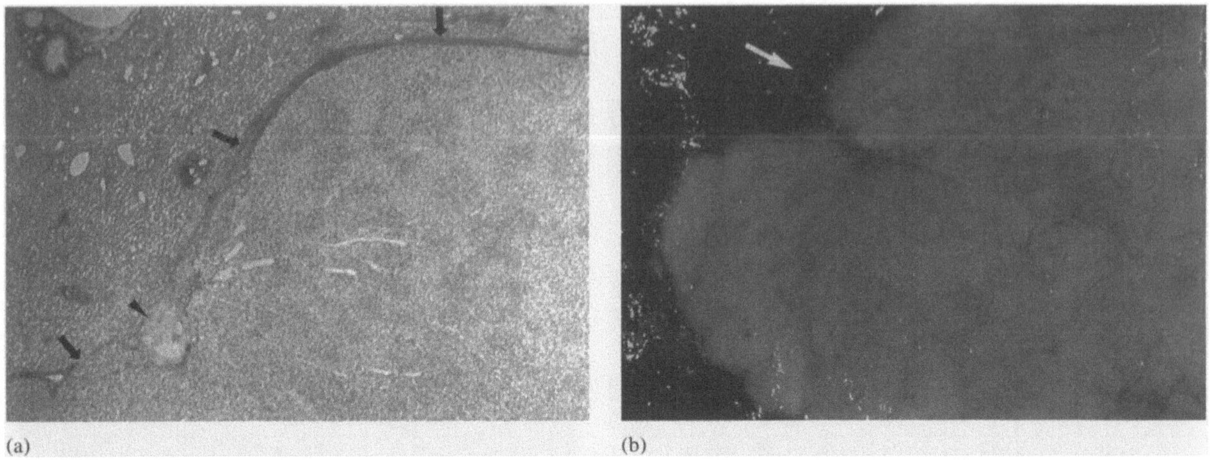


**Figure 8.5** Hepatocellular adenoma (HCA). **a**. Low-power H&E photomicrograph reveals a fibrous capsule surrounding the lesion (straight arrows) with a subcapsular vessel (arrowhead). Note the paler HCA compared with normal liver due to high fat contents. **b**. Cut section demonstrates a mosaic appearance of fat and cellular HCA in this lesion with a well-defined border. A large capsular vessel is noted (arrow)

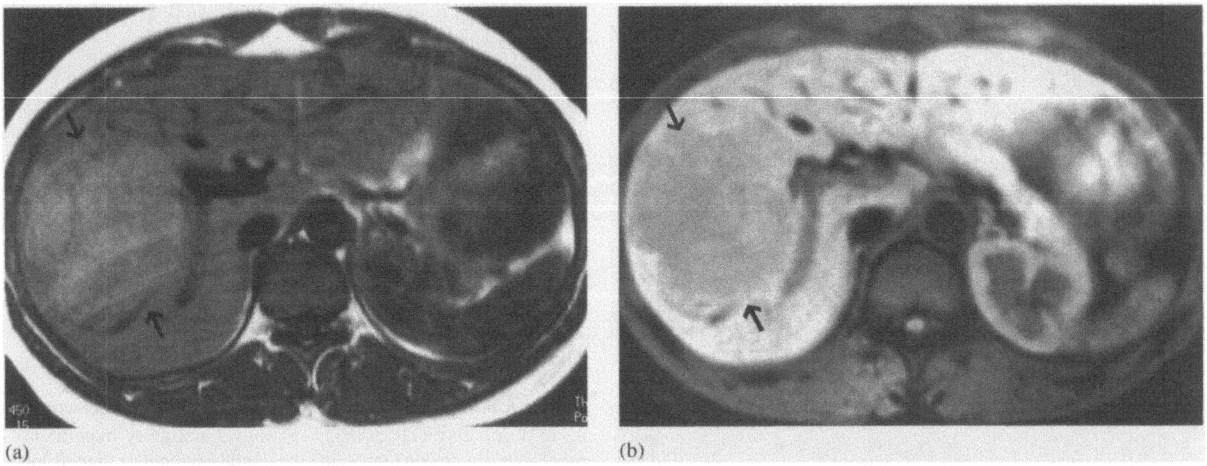


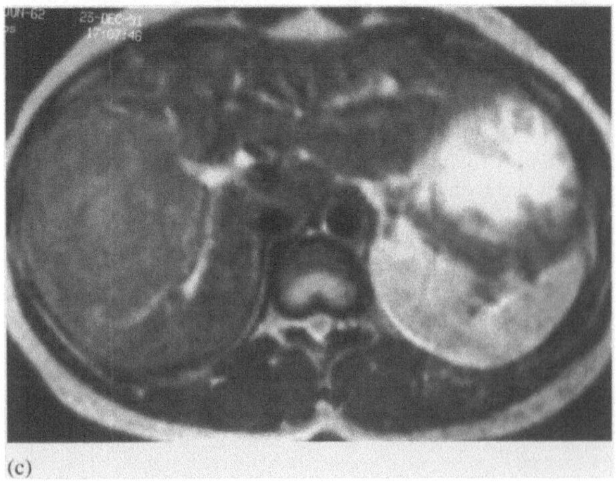


**Figure 8.6** Hepatocellular adenoma in a 29-year-old woman. **a**. T1W imaging (TR 450/TE 15) shows a mass (arrows) in the right lobe of the liver to have slightly increased signal intensity relative to the liver. **b**. Fat suppression T1W imaging (TR 550/TE 15) now demonstrates the lesion (arrows) to be hypointense to the liver, indicating its fatty nature. **c**. T2W imaging (TR 2000/TE 90) shows the mass to be slightly hyperintense

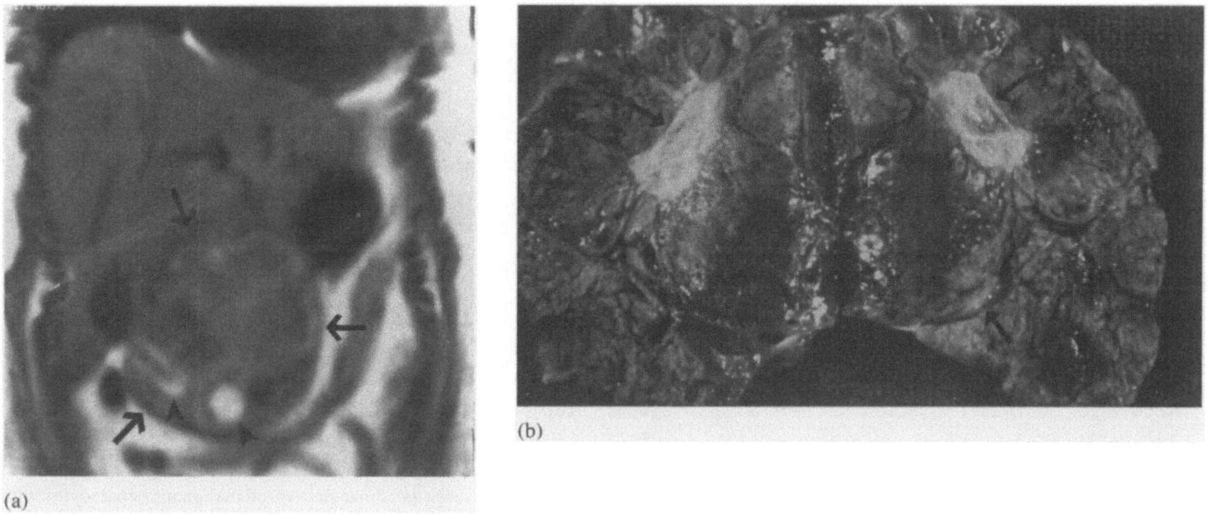

Figure 8.7 Hepatocellular adenoma in a 25-year-old woman. a. Coronal T1W imaging (TR 450/TE 15) shows a large exophytic mass (arrows) containing hyperintense areas which corresponded to haemorrhage (arrowheads). b. Cut gross specimen demonstrates areas of fibrosis (arrows), haemorrhage and fat

**Table 8.3 Hepatocellular adenoma: MRI–pathological correlation**

| *Pathology features* | *MRI appearance* |
|---|---|
| • Large tumour usually surrounded by a capsule containing multiple large vessels | • Large lesion with multiple surrounding vessels |
| • Contains haemorrhage and infarction commonly | • Heterogeneous appearance on T1W and T2W imaging |
| • Rich in fat | • Hyperintense in T1W imaging; hypointense in fat-suppressed images |
| • Contains Kupffer cells, but poor vascularity | • Poor SPIO uptake |

sis due to alcohol abuse, haemochromatosis, toxin exposure or hepatitis is responsible. Serum $\alpha$-fetoprotein levels are usually markedly elevated.

Histologically, malignant hepatocytes are present in HCC (Figure 8.8a). The malignant hepatocytes may be so well differentiated that bile may be produced (Figure 8.8a). The cytoplasm of HCC hepatocytes may contain fat and glycogen[7]. It may be difficult to differentiate the cells of HCC from normal hepatocytes and/or hepatocellular adenoma, which may affect the accuracy of fine-needle aspiration biopsy.

Grossly, considerable variation occurs, with solitary, multifocal and diffuse growth patterns described. A variant of the solitary form, encapsulated HCC, may have an improved prognosis due to increased resectability[22]. Vascular invasion of hepatic veins, inferior vena cava (IVC) and portal vein is common. Frequently, internal necrosis and haemorrhage are present due to the tumour's lack of stroma (Figure 8.8b).

### *MR imaging*

HCC has a variable MR imaging appearance depending upon its growth pattern. Vascular invasion is well displayed if present, particularly using gradient-echo images[1].

On T1W imaging, HCC varies in appearance from hypointense to hyperintense depending upon the

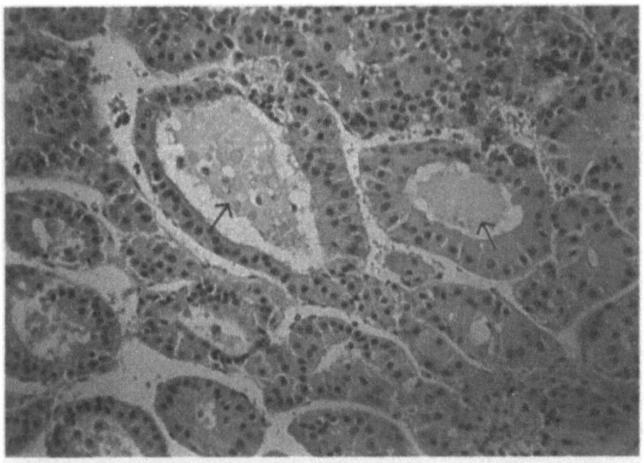
(a)

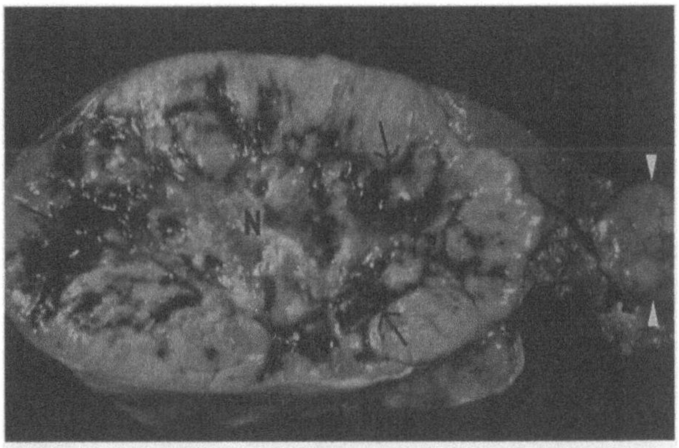

(b)

**Figure 8.8** Hepatocellular carcinoma. **a**. High power H&E photomicrograph reveals an acinar pattern of malignant hepatocytes with pseudogland formation. Bile production is present (arrows). This acinar pattern with high aqueous contents results in heterogeneous hyperintensity on T2W imaging. **b**. This gross specimen demonstrates central necrosis (N) with areas of haemorrhage (arrows). A satellite lesion is nearby (arrowheads)

**Table 8.4 Hepatocellular carcinoma: MRI-pathological correlation**

| *Pathology features* | *MRI appearance* |
|---|---|
| • Solitary, multifocal and diffuse growth patterns | • Solitary and multifocal masses well depicted; diffuse lesion detection may be difficult |
| • Encapsulated form has fibrous capsule | • Hypointense peripheral rim |
| • Fatty change | • Increased signal intensity on T1W imaging; decreased signal intensity well-defined margins on fat-suppressed images |
| • Fibrosis | • Isointense areas on T1W and T2W imaging |
| • Necrosis | • Hypointense T1W and T2W imaging |
| • Haemorrhage | • Hypointense T1W and T2W imaging; marked hyperintensity in fat-suppressed images |
| • Vascular invasion | • Abnormal signal in vessels on T1W and T2W imaging, flow abnormalities on gradient-echo imaging |
| • Malignant hepatocytes | • No uptake of iv SPIO |

presence or absence of steatosis and/or areas of haemorrhage[24]. On T2W imaging, the lesions may have mild hyperintensity relative to normal liver with increased signal intensity seen in areas of necrosis[25,26] (Figure 8.9a).

The encapsulated form of HCC often has a low signal rim, representing the tumour capsule[26].

After the iv administration of Gd-DTPA, there is usually enhancement of its non-necrotic areas that are hypervascular[11]. After iv SPIO, there is improved lesion detectability, especially of small satellite lesions, due to the decreased signal intensity of non-involved liver[5,27] (Figure 8.9), while HCC remains hyperintense due to lack of SPIO uptake (Table 8.4).

## Fibrolamellar carcinoma

### *Pathology*

Fibrolamellar carcinoma (FLC) is a slow-growing hepatocellular carcinoma occurring primarily in young adults[7]. The mean survival is better than that of HCC, with FLC having an improved likelihood of cure (40%) if surgically resected.

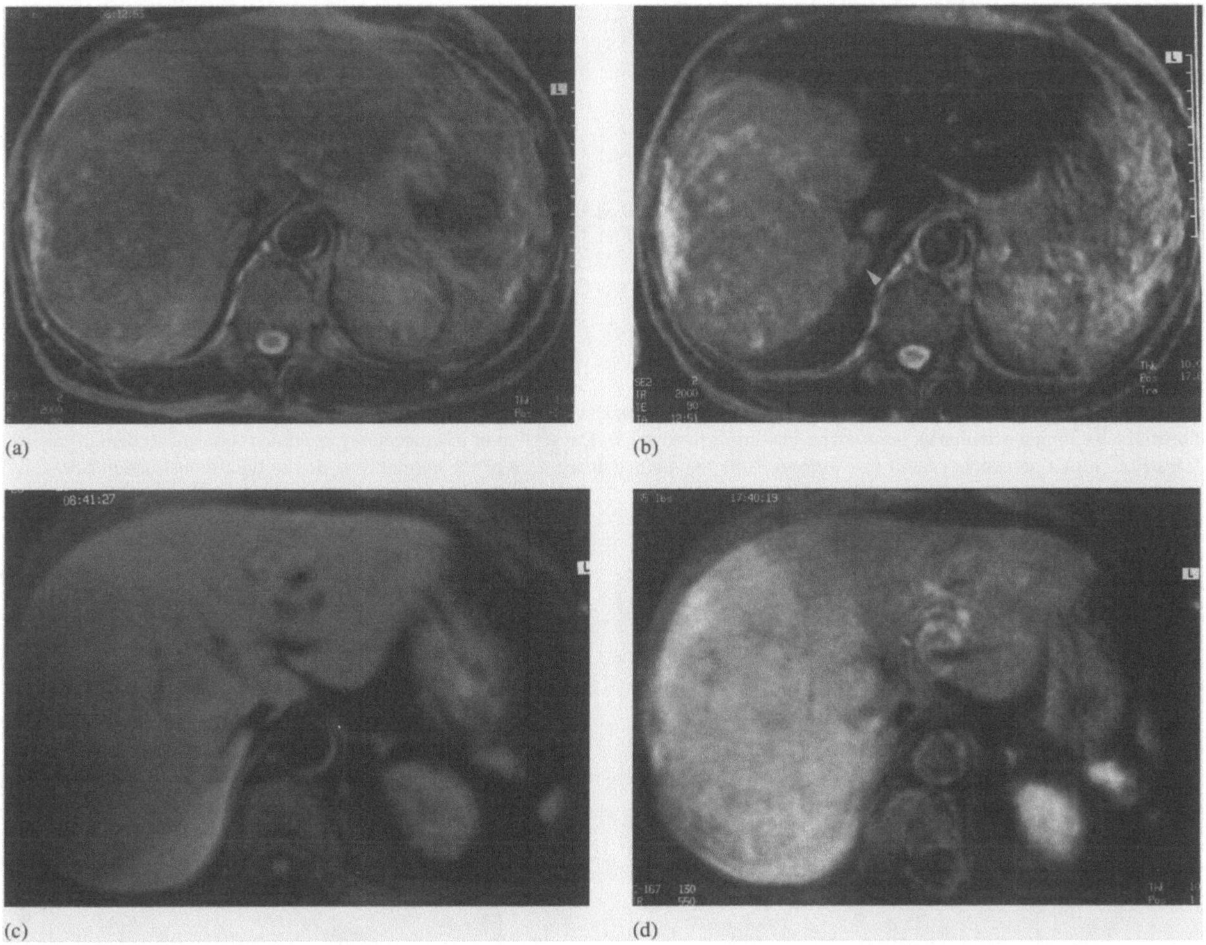

(a) (b) (c) (d)

**Figure 8.9** Hepatocellular carcinoma in a 63-year-old cirrhotic man. **a.** T2W imaging (TR 2000/TE 90) demonstrates slightly increased heterogeneous signal intensity involving the right lobe of the liver. A mass is not clearly seen. **b.** Post-iv SPIO imaging (TR 2000/TE 90). A large lesion is now well defined as increased signal while the normal liver demonstrates marked signal decrease. A small satellite lesion is also revealed (arrowhead). **c.** Fat-suppression pre-iv SPIO T1W imaging shows the mass to have slightly decreased signal relative to the remainder of the liver. **d.** Post-iv SPIO fat suppression T1W imaging demonstrates improved conspicuity of the lesion when compared with **c**

Histologically, malignant hepatocytes are separated into cords by strands of lamellar fibrosis (Figure 8.10a). There are no $\alpha$-fetoprotein body inclusions, unlike in HCC[7].

Grossly, FLC is a large solitary homogeneous mass which may be pedunculated. It often has a central fibrous scar with multiple fibrous septa, similar in appearance to FNH[7] (Figure 8.10b) except for possible calcifications. The tumour is well demarcated from the usually normal surrounding liver, and satellite nodules may occur. Haemorrhage and necrosis are rarely seen in FLC.

*MR imaging*

On T1W imaging, the lesion is isointense relative to normal liver[14,28] (Figure 8.11a). On T2W imaging, FLC is also usually isointense relative to normal liver, although it has been reported as slightly hyperintense or hypointense[28] (Figure 8.11b). If pre-

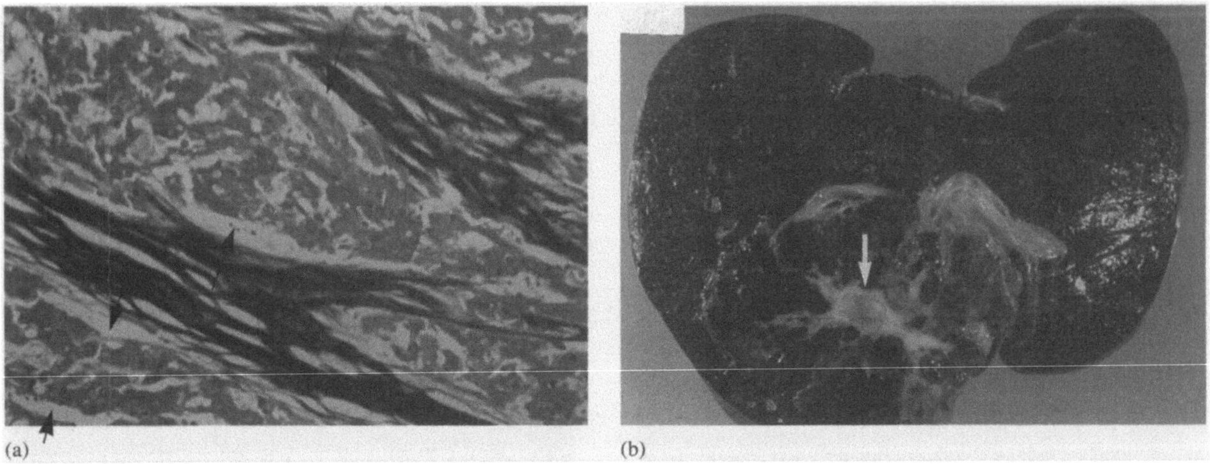

**Figure 8.10** Fibrolamellar carcinoma (FLC). **a** Low-power Masson-stain photomicrograph reveals the dark-staining bands of lamellar fibrosis, separating the malignant hepatocytes into cords (arrows). **b**. Cut section of a hepatectomy specimen (transplant) demonstrates a large FLC with a prominent central scar (arrow). Note the nutmeg appearance of the normal liver due to biliary obstruction caused by tumour.

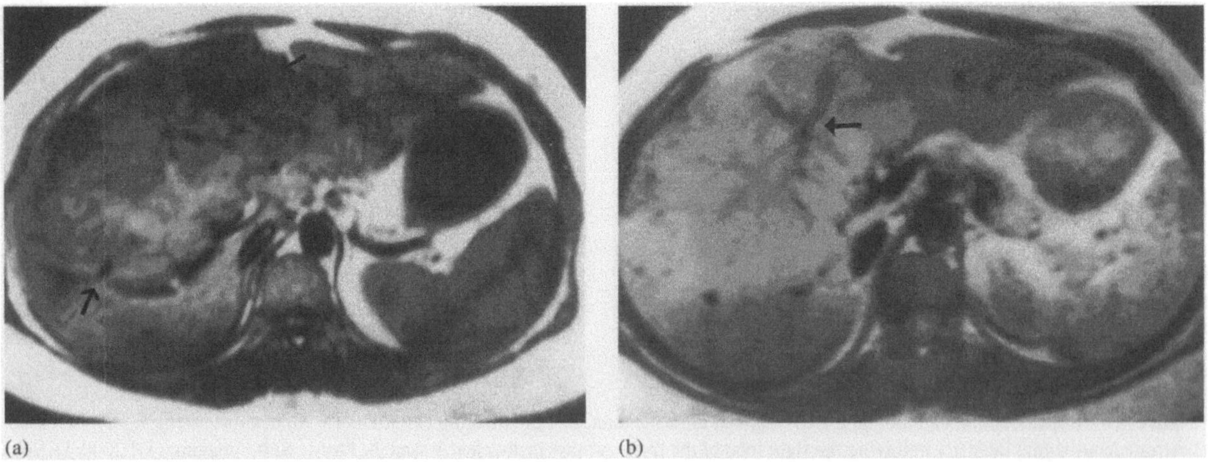

**Figure 8.11** Fibrolamellar carcinoma. **a**. T1W imaging demonstrates a large mass (arrows) which is isointense to the normal liver. **b**. T2W imaging shows the mass to be mildly hyperintense to the liver. The fibrous scar remains hypointense, unlike in FNH where the central scar is frequently hyperintense in T2W imaging

sent, the central fibrous scar is hypointense on both T1W imaging and T2W imaging due to its fibrous nature and/or calcification. This hypointensity of the central scar of FLC may be useful for distinguishing it from the hyperintense central scar of FNH in T2W imaging[14] (Table 8.5).

## Intrahepatic cholangiocarcinoma

*Pathology*

Intrahepatic cholangiocarcinoma (I-CAC) is an uncommon primary liver malignancy (compared with HCC), occurring in patients with an average age of 50–60 years with a slight male predominance[30]. Jaundice is rare as I-CAC arises in peripheral bile ducts, unlike the more common extrahepatic cholangiocarcinoma where jaundice is common[7].

Histologically, I-CAC is an adenocarcinoma arising from the epithelium of an intrahepatic bile duct (Figure 8.12a). Desmoplastic reaction is often prominent, as well as mucin production and intratumoural calcification[7].

Grossly, I-CAC is a large firm homogeneous mass with predominantly whitish fibrous stroma (Figure 8.12b). It may have small areas of necrosis or haemorrhage. Encasement without invasion of large vessels is common.

*MR imaging*

I-CAC appears by MR imaging as a large central mass, which encases large vessels, such as the portal vein, hepatic veins or IVC, but without tumour thrombus (Figure 8.13). On T1W imaging, it is hypointense[29], and, on T2W imaging, the periphery is hyperintense relative to normal liver, while large central fibrosis

**Table 8.5 Fibrolamellar carcinoma: MRI–pathological correlation**

| *Pathology features* | *MRI appearance* |
|---|---|
| • Homogeneous tumour of malignant hepatocytes | • Homogeneous appearance of mild hypointensity on T1W imaging and slight hyperintensity on T2W imaging |
| • Central scar of lamellar fibrosis | • Hypointense central scar on T1W and T2W imaging |

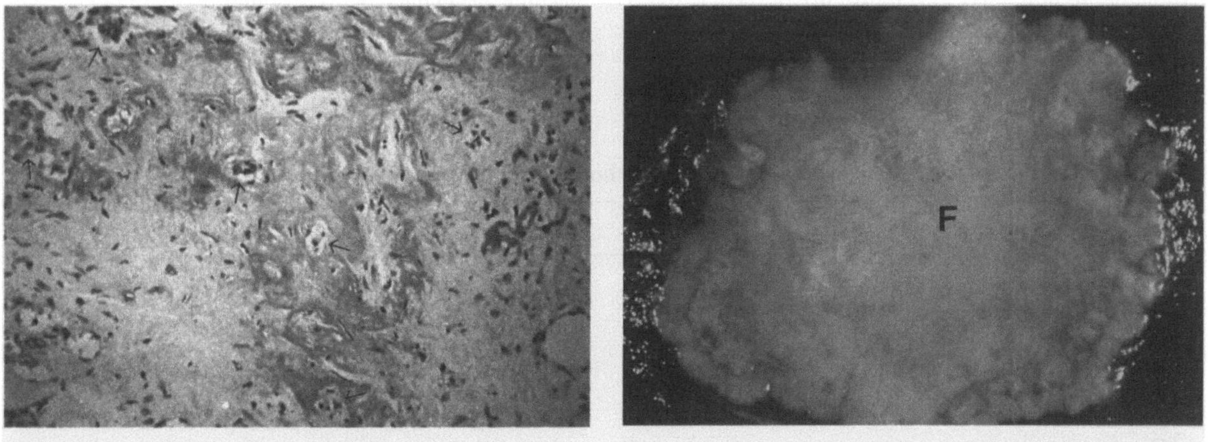


(a) (b)

**Figure 8.12** Intrahepatic cholangiocarcinoma (I-CAC). **a.** High-power H&E photomicrograph reveals glandular malignant cells (arrows) interspersed in a magna of fibrous tissue, typical of I-CAC. **b.** Cut section shows a large area of central fibrosis (F) within the centre of this large I-CAC. Note the lobulated contour of the mass

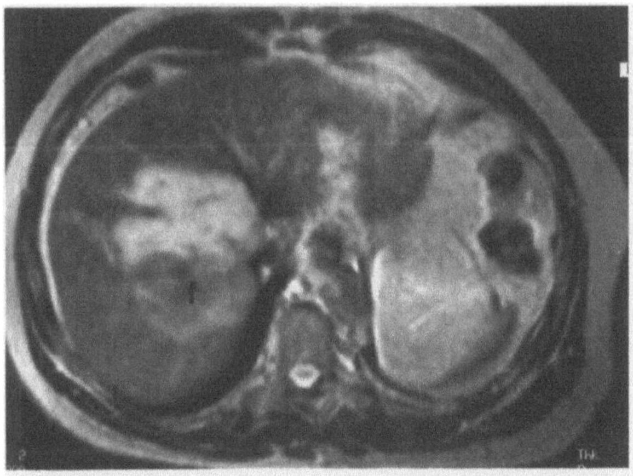

(a)

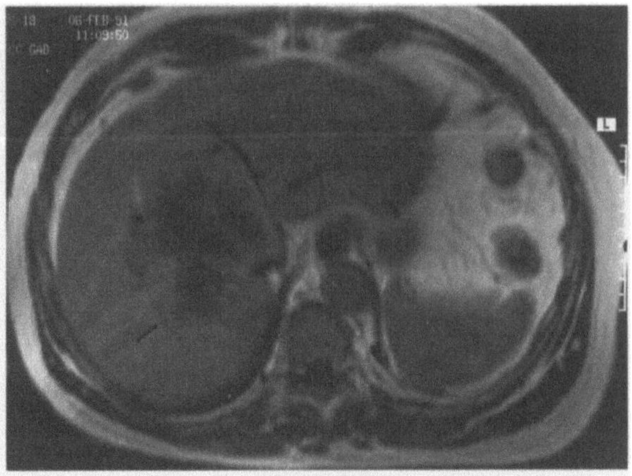

(b)

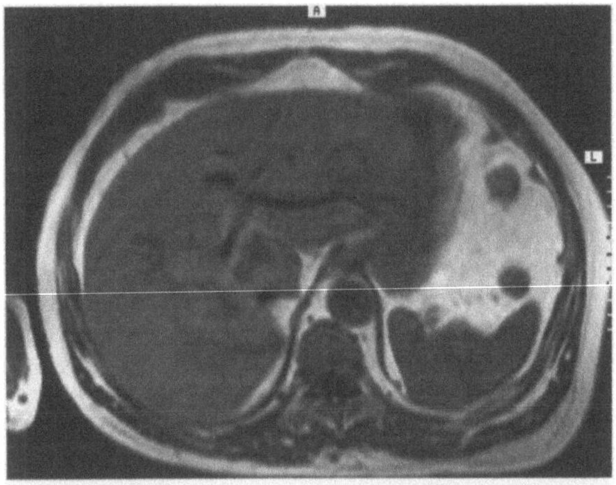

(c)

**Figure 8.13** Intrahepatic cholangiocarcinoma in a 72-year-old man. **a**. T2W imaging (TR 2000/TE 90) demonstrates a predominantly increased signal intensity lesion with central decreased signal intensity (f) representing fibrosis. Note the well-defined and lobulated contour, correlating with 8.12b. **b**. T1W imaging (TR 303/TE 15) obtained immediately after iv Gd-DTPA shows centripetal enhancement of the predominantly hypointense lesion. A non-enhancing hypointense rim defines a portion of the perimeter of the mass (arrow). **c**. Delayed T1W imaging (TR 303/TE 15) (obtained several minutes post-Gd-DTPA injection) shows centripetal enhancement of the I-CAC compared with **b**. Note the encased but patent right portal vein and IVC

remains hypointense[28] (Figure 8.13). After the iv administration of Gd-DTPA, a pattern of progressive concentric enhancement is seen due to peripheral cellular tumour (marked enhancement) versus central fibrosis (sparse enhancement) (Figure 8.13b). Gradient-echo imaging and MR angiography demonstrate well the characteristic finding of I-CAC of vascular encasement without tumour thrombus (Table 8.6).

**Table 8.6 Intrahepatic cholangiocarcinoma: MRI–pathological correlation**

| *Pathology features* | *MRI appearance* |
|---|---|
| • Large firm mass with little haemorrhage or necrosis | • Homogeneous appearance with low signal intensity on T1W imaging |
| • Periphery of tumour is more viable | • Hyperintense peripheral regions on T2W imaging |
| • Central fibrosis | • Low signal intensity centrally on T2W imaging |
| • Vascular encasement without invasion | • No evidence of tumour thrombus |

## Biliary cystadenoma/cystadenocarcinoma

### *Pathology*

Biliary cystadenoma is an uncommon cystic multilocular intrahepatic tumour occurring in adults, most commonly middle-aged women. Recurrence following resection of cystadenoma is common, with malignant transformation to cystadenocarcinoma often occurring over several years[7].

Histologically, the locules are lined by either benign or malignant biliary type epithelial cells in cystadenoma or cystadenocarcinoma, respectively (Figure 8.14a). Focal calcifications within the wall can be present. Cystadenoma and cystadenocarcinoma are seen as two extremes of the same lesion. Therefore, all cystadenomas are considered as premalignant and with potential for malignant recurrence[7,31].

Grossly, cystadenoma/cystadenocarcinoma is usually a large multilocular intrahepatic cystic mass containing proteinaceous fluid[32]. Dense solid polypoid masses on the internal wall indicate a malignant component. However, papillary areas and polypoid projections are seen in cystadenoma without frank malignancy (Figure 8.14b).

### *MR imaging*

Cystadenoma/cystadenocarcinoma appear on MR imaging as large multilocular intrahepatic cystic lesions which may have an irregular wall[32]. On T1W imaging, there is variable signal intensity of the locules depending upon their protein content[32] (Figure 8.15a). This may be of help in distinguishing cystadenoma/cystadenocarcinoma from other cystic masses, such as complicated cysts or bilomas. On T2W imaging, the lesion is hyperintense relative to normal liver but of varied signal intensity depending upon protein content of locules[32] (Figure 8.15b). Although solid components are more often seen with cystadenocarcinoma, the only reliable signs of malignancy are the presence of adenopathy or metastatic disease (Table 8.7).

## Conclusion

MR imaging is developing as a powerful modality in the evaluation of focal liver lesions, particularly primary neoplasms. Through the use of standard spin-echo techniques, as well as advanced sequences and contrast agents, tissue characterization has improved, since MR imaging provides not only anatomical detail but also physiological information. The correlation between the underlying key pathological features of primary hepatic tumours with their often complex MR appearances, leads to a better understanding of these tumours.

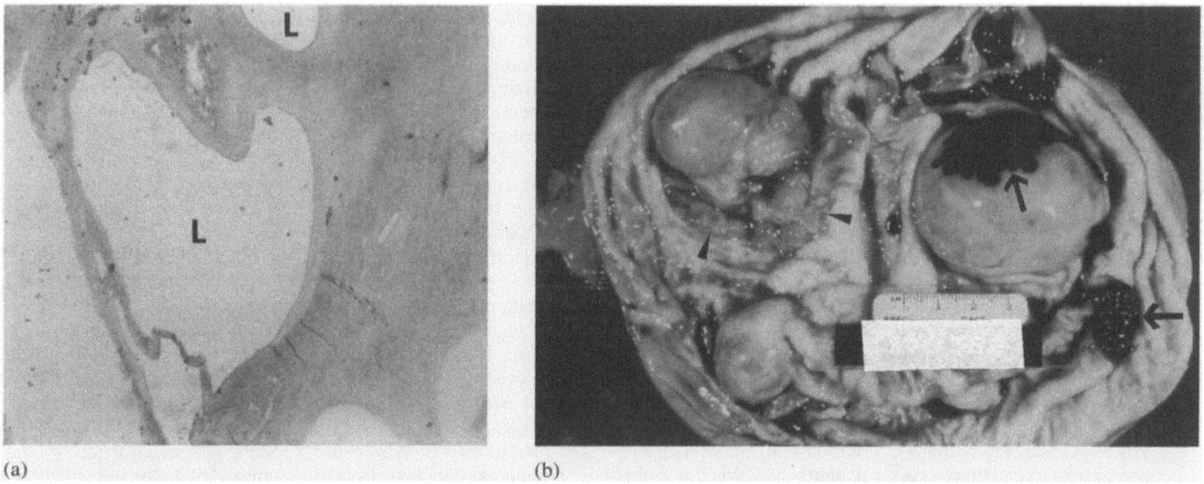


**Figure 8.14** Biliary cystadenoma. **a**. Low-power H&E photomicrograph demonstrates the locules (L), which contain the proteinaceous tumoural secretions, lined with biliary epithelium and surrounded by solid areas. **b**. The glistening surface of this gross specimen is covered by haemorrhage in several areas (straight arrows). Mural nodules are present (arrowheads)

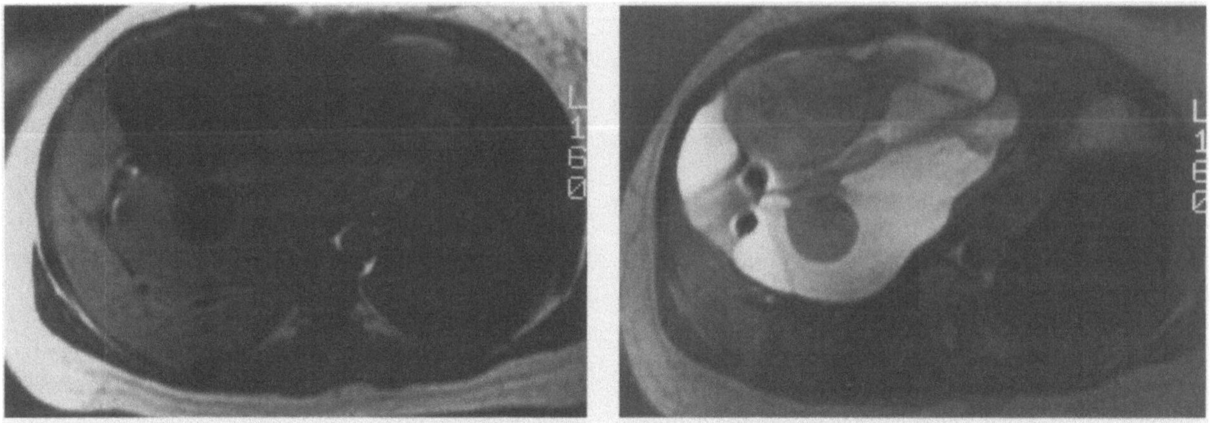

(a) (b)

**Figure 8.15** Recurrent cystadenoma in a 37-year-old woman. **a.** On T1W imaging (TR 500/TE 20), a large intrahepatic mass composed of multiple locules of variable hypointense signal intensity is seen. Metal artifact is seen in the periphery of the mass (right) due to clips from prior resection. **b.** T2W imaging (TR 2200/TE 80) shows different intensities in the locules, corresponding to variable degree of proteinaceous contents (i.e. blood products, bile, etc.). Variable intensities in a multiloculated cystic mass suggests neoplasm, such as cystadenoma/cystadenocarcinoma

**Table 8.7 Biliary cystadenoma/cystadenocarcinoma: MRI–pathological correlation**

| *Pathology features* | *MRI appearance* |
|---|---|
| • Large multiloculated intrahepatic cyst | • Large, multilocular lesion |
| • Contains proteinaceous fluid of varying concentrations | • Variable signal intensity on T1W imaging and variable hyperintense signal intensity on T2W imaging |

*Acknowledgements*

The author thanks all radiologists and pathologists who have submitted their case to the Armed Forces Institute of Pathology as some of their material is included in this article. Thanks are also due to Cathryn Powers MD, former Fellow at the University of Florida, for her contributions which resulted in an exhibit based on this review, and to Ms Linda Pigott for her assistance in the preparation of this manuscript.

*References*

1. Powers C, Ros PR, Stoupis C, Johnson WK, Segel K. Liver neoplasms: magnetic resonance imaging–pathologic correlation. RadioGraphics 1994;14:459–482.
2. Bydder GM, Steiner RE, Blumgart LH, et al. MR imaging of the liver using short T1 inversion recovery sequences. J Comput Assist Tomogr. 1985;9(6):1084–9.
3. Egglin TK, Rummeney E, Stark DD, et al. Hepatic tumors: quantitative tissue characterization with MR imaging. Radiology. 1990;176:107–10.
4. Hamm B, Fischer E, Taupitz M. Differentiation of hepatic hemangiomas from metastases by dynamic contrast-enhanced MR imaging. J Comput Assist Tomogr. 1990; 14(2):205–16.
5. Ferrucci JT, Stark DD. Iron oxide-enhanced MR imaging of the liver and spleen: review of the first 5 years. Am J Roentgenol. 1990;155:943–50.
6. Hamm B, Vogel TJ, Branding G, et al. Focal liver lesions: MR imaging with Mn-DPDP – initial clinical results in 40 patients. Radiology. 1922;182:167–74.
7. Craig JR, Peters RL, Edmondson HA. Tumors of the liver and intrahepatic bile ducts. In: Craig JR, Peters RC, Edmondson HA, eds. Atlas of tumor pathology. Washington, DC: Armed Forces Institute of Pathology; 1989.
8. Rummeny E, Weissleder R, Stark DD, et al. Primary liver tumors: diagnosis by MR imaging. Am J Roentgenol. 1989; 152:63–72.
9. Ros PR, Lubbers PR, Olmsted WW, et al. Hemangioma of the liver: heterogeneous appearance on T2-weighted images. Am J Roentganol. 1987;149:1167–70.

10. Stark DD, Felder RC, Wittenberg J, et al. Magnetic resonance imaging of cavernous hemangioma of the liver: tissue-specific characterization. Am J Roentgenol. 1985; 145:213–22.
11. Bree RL, Schwab RE, Glazer GM, et al. The varied appearances of hepatic cavernous hemangiomas with sonography, computed tomography, magnetic resonance imaging and scintigraphy. RadioGraphics. 1987;7:1153–75.
12. Yoshida H, Itai Y, Ohtomo K, et al. Small hepatocellular carcinoma and cavernous hemangioma: differentiation with dynamic FLASH MR imaging with Gd-DTPA. Radiology. 1989;171:339–42.
13. Wanless IR, Mawdsley C, Adams R. Pathogenesis of focal nodular hyperplasia. Hepatology. 1985;5:1194–1200.
14. Mattison GR, Glazer GM, Quint LE, et al. MR imaging of hepatic focal nodular hyperplasia: characterization and distinction from primary malignant hepatic tumors. Am J Roentgenol. 1987;148:711–15.
15. Butch RJ, Stark DD, Malt RA. MR imaging of hepatic focal nodular hyperplasia. J Comput Assist Tomogr. 1986;10:874–7.
16. Rummeny E, Weissleder R, Sironi S, et al. Central scars in primary liver tumors: MR features, specificity, and pathologic correlation. Radiology. 1989;171:323–6.
17. Schiebler ML, Kressel HY, Saul SH, et al. MR imaging of focal nodular hyperplasia of the liver. J Comput Assist Tomogr. 1987;11:651–4.
18. Christopherson WM, Mays ET, Barrows G. A clinicopathologic study of steroid-related tumors. Am J Surg Pathol. 1977;1:31–41.
19. Goodman ZD, et al. Kupffer cells in hepatocellular adenomas. Am J Surg Pathol. 1987;11:191–6.
20. Gabata T, Matsui O, Kadoya M, et al. MR imaging of hepatic adenoma. Am J Roentgenol. 1990;155:1009–11.
21. Nokes SR, Baker ME, Spritzer CE, et al. Hepatic adenoma: MR appearance mimicking focal nodular hyperplasia. J Comput Assist Tomogr. 1988;12:885–7.
22. Freeney PC, Baron RL, Teefey SA. Hepatocellular carcinoma: reduced frequency of typical findings with dynamic contrast-enhanced CT in a non-Asian population. Radiology. 1992;182:143–8.
23. Itoh K, Nishimura K, Togashi K, et al. Hepatocellular carcinoma: MR imaging. Radiology. 1987;164:21–5.
24. Moss AA, Goldberg HJ, Stark DD, et al. Hepatic tumors: magnetic resonance and CT appearance. Radiology. 1984; 150:141–7.
25. Ohtomo K, Itai Y, Furui S, et al. Hepatic tumors: differentiation by transverse relaxation time (T2) of magnetic resonance imaging. Radiology. 1985;155:421–3.
26. Ros PR, et al. Encapsulated hepatocellular carcinoma: radiologic findings and pathologic correlation. Gastrointest Radiol. 1990;15:233–7.
27. Fretz CJ, Elizondo G, Weissleder R, et al. Superparamagnetic iron oxide-enhanced MR imaging: pulse sequence optimization for detection of liver cancer. Radiology. 1989;172:393–7.
28. Titelbaum DS, Hatabu H, Schiebler ML, et al. Fibrolamellar hepatocellular carcinoma: MR appearance. J Comput Assist Tomogr. 1988;12(4):588–91.
29. Hamrick-Turner J, Abbitt PL, Ros PR. Intrahepatic cholangiocarcinoma: MR appearance. Am J Roentgenol. 1992; 158:77–9.
30. O'Neil J, Ros PR. Knowing hepatic pathology aids MRI of liver tumors. Diagn Imaging. 1989;Dec:58–67.
31. Ishak KG, et al. Biliary cystadenoma and cystadenocarcinoma. Cancer. 1977;38:322–38.
32. Palacios E, Shannon M, Solomon C, et al. Biliary cystadenoma: ultrasound, CT and MRI. Gastrointest Radiol. 1990; 15:313–16.

# 9

# USE OF CONTRAST AGENTS IN THE DETECTION AND DIFFERENTIATION OF FOCAL LIVER LESIONS BY MR IMAGING: Gd-DTPA, Mn-DPDP AND IRON OXIDE

B. HAMM AND M. TAUPITZ

## Introduction

MR imaging has a higher sensitivity in the detection of focal liver lesions than CT[1–3]. Of particular interest is a paper published by Heiken and co-workers[4], who compared the sensitivities of contrast-enhanced CT, CT during arterial portography (CTAP) and MR imaging, and correlated the results with histopathological findings. The highest sensitivity was found for CTAP (81%), followed by MR imaging (57%) and contrast-enhanced CT (38%). The rather high error rates of MR imaging and contrast-enhanced CT were due to the poor visualization of small metastases with a diameter of less than 1 cm. Since, however, CTAP is a complex and invasive procedure, research in this area is aimed at improving the sensitivity of liver MR imaging by new technical developments and by the use of tissue-specific contrast agents. MR imaging has a remarkably high diagnostic accuracy in the differentiation of liver tumours, since the information displayed on MR images is far superior to that obtained by ultrasound or CT. In the clinical setting, this advantage of MR imaging is of particular importance in differentiating haemangiomas and metastases – the most frequent benign and malignant tumours of the liver[5–7].

## Contrast agents for liver MR imaging

A general aim of contrast application is to improve image contrast. Contrast agents used in the detection of focal liver lesions should therefore selectively alter the signal intensity of either of the two tissue – normal liver parenchyma or focal lesion. Substances with these properties are so-called tissue-specific contrast agents. In addition, contrast agents should permit the differentiation of benign from malignant liver lesions and also reduce the examination time per patient. The contrast agents already being used in clinical studies of liver MR imaging can be subdivided into three groups:

1. Contrast agents of the extracellular space,
2. Superparamagnetic iron oxide particles taken up by the reticuloendothelial system, and
3. Hepatobiliary contrast agents.

### *Contrast agents of the extracellular space*

Gadolinium compounds with distribution in the extracellular space have pharmacokinetic properties comparable to those of iodinated contrast agents used in X-ray examinations. Diagnostically adequate images are obtained by combining fast MR imaging with bolus application of the contrast agent. Optimal contrast between hypovascularized solid tumours and liver tissue occurs about 15–150 seconds after injection of Gd-DTPA[9]. Given the fact that the imaging window is short and tissue-specific contrast agents will soon be available, contrast agents of the extracellular space will probably not play a role in the detection of liver lesions. However, Gd-DTPA-enhanced dynamic MR examinations have some significance in the differentiation of hepatic tumours[10–13]. In dynamic MR imaging, liver haemangiomas are characterized by the well-known fill-in phenomenon and a high signal intensity in the delayed phase (about 10 minutes after contrast application), while metastases show inhomogeneous contrast enhancement and do not become isointense to the surrounding liver parenchyma. Dynamic MR imaging is a highly suitable modality for differentiating haemangiomas from metastases in cases where non-enhanced T2 weighted images to do not allow a clear distinction. Hepatocellular carcinomas may be either hypovascularized or hypervascularized and thus show only slight or very strong contrast enhancement, which is typically inhomogeneous. The peritumoural pseudocapsule of a hepatocellular carcinoma displays late contrast enhancement after several minutes. Dynamic MR imaging is especially useful in diagnosing focal nodular hyperplasia. We studied the contrast behaviour of this benign tumour in dynamic MR imaging in a recently completed study of 48 cases of focal nodular hyperplasia performed at Steglitz Medical Center of the Free University of Berlin and at the Charité of Humboldt University (unpublished data). All focal nodular hyperplasias showed strong and early contrast enhancement, which was homogeneous in 92% of the cases. 64% of the lesions had a central scar with delayed enhancement after 2–4 minutes (Figure 9.1). The question that arises here is whether dynamic MR imaging is at all able to distinguish benign and malignant hypervascularized liver tumours. A recent study including 28 focal nodular hyperplasias and 22 hypervascularized malignant tumours (e.g. carcinoid metastases, hepatocellular carcinomas) demonstrated that malignant tumours can also show early enhancement, but the pattern is never homogeneous and the central scar is typically absent[14].

The improved differentiation of focal liver lesions by dynamic MR imaging found in the first clinical trial

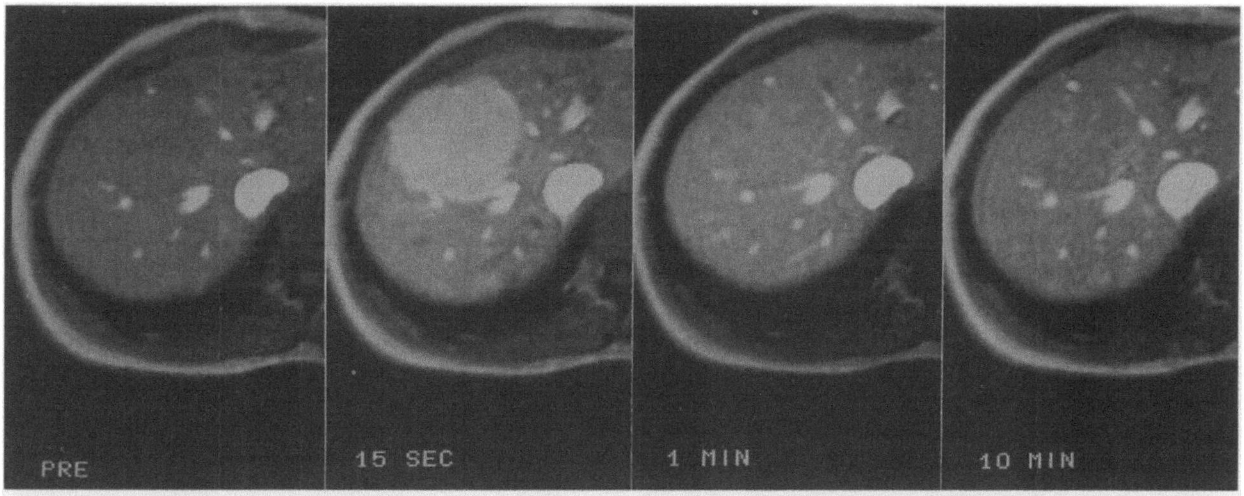


(a) (b) (c) (d)

**Figure 9.1** Dynamic Gd-DTPA-enhanced MR imaging of a focal nodular hyperplasia (0.1 mmol Gd-DTPA/kg; GRE 100/5/80°). Note the strong and homogeneous enhancement of the lesion. **a** Precontrast; **b** 15 s postcontrast; **c** 1 min postcontrast; **d** 10 min postcontrast

was re-evaluated in a prospective study including 107 patients. All patients underwent MR imaging according to an identical protocol, and the images were then randomized and evluated independently by four experienced radiologists without knowledge of clinical data. In this study, the combined non-enhanced and dynamic MR images significantly improved the differentiation of benign and malignant liver tumours compared with non-enhanced images alone[15].

### *Superparamagnetic iron oxide particles*

Superparamagnetic iron oxide particles are taken up by the cells of the reticuloendothelial system (RES)

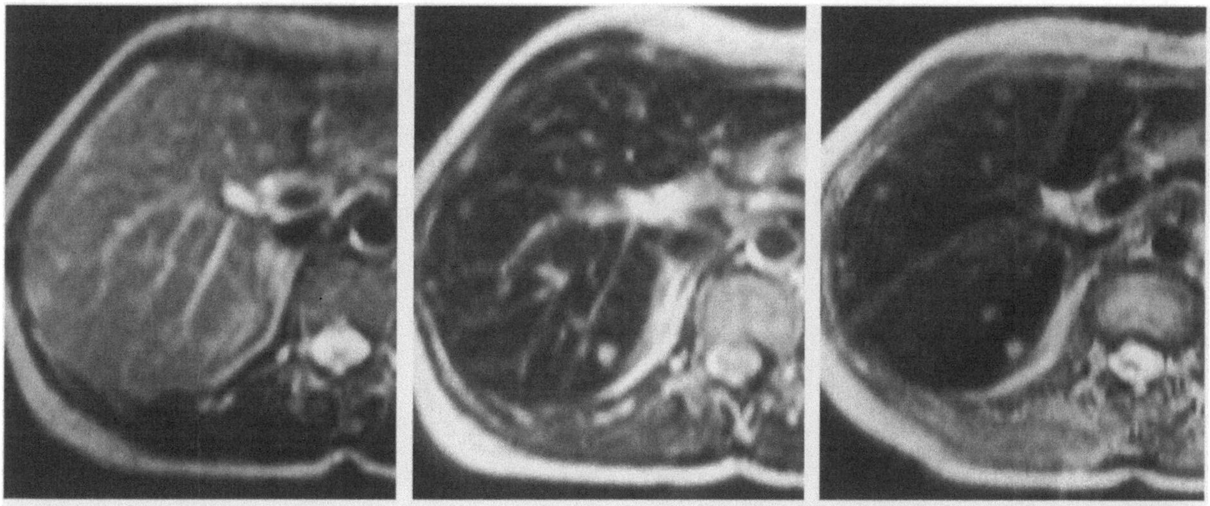

(a) (b) (c)

**Figure 9.2** Liver metastases from a carcinoid before (**a**, SE 2300/90) and after (**b**, SE 2300/45; **c**, PSIF 10/18/15°) intravenous application of iron oxide (AMI-25, 15 $\mu$mol Fe/kg). Compared with the precontrast T2 weighted image (**a**), there is an improved lesion-to-liver contrast after intravenous application of IOP (**b**). Small lesions and intrahepatic vessels appear bright on the conventional SE postcontrast image. An increased number of small lesions can be detected after contrast application by using the PSIF sequence (**c**), which led to a signal void in the intrahepatic vessels and thus produce a pronounced signal reduction in liver parenchyma, while the signal intensity of metastases, which do not have an RES, is not affected by the contrast material. This difference results in a markedly enhanced contrast between liver and tumour compared with non-enhanced images. The sensitivity of this contrast agent in the detection of liver metastases has been reported to differ for intermediate and high magnetic field strengths[16,17]. At an intermediate field strength (approx. 0.6 Tesla), Stark and co-workers found a significantly increased tumour/liver contrast after intravenous application of superparamagnetic iron oxide particles and detected significantly more liver lesions than on non-enhanced images[17]. At high magnetic field strength (1.5 Tesla), Marchal and co-workers also found tumour/liver contrast to be improved after contrast application, but the number of lesions detected did not differ significantly from that already identified on T2 weighted precontrast images[16]. The effect of AMI-25 as a superparamagnetic contrast agent is currently being investigated in a European multicentre study. Preliminary results of this study suggest that superparamagnetic iron oxide

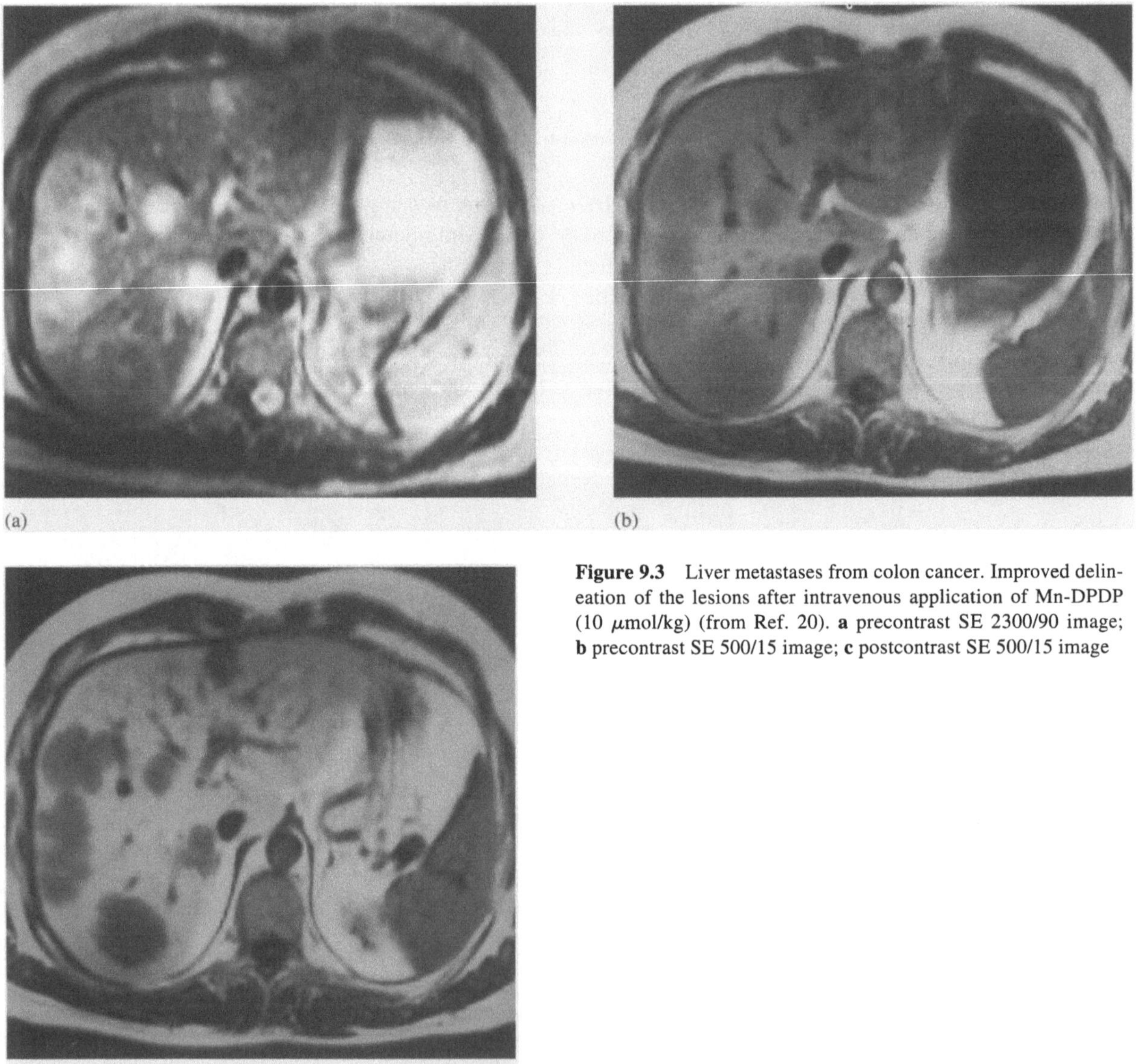

(a) (b) (c)

**Figure 9.3** Liver metastases from colon cancer. Improved delineation of the lesions after intravenous application of Mn-DPDP (10 μmol/kg) (from Ref. 20). **a** precontrast SE 2300/90 image; **b** precontrast SE 500/15 image; **c** postcontrast SE 500/15 image particles also improve the detection of liver metastases at high magnetic field strengths when used in combination with new optimized pulse sequences[18] (Figure 9.2).

### *Hepatobiliary contrast agents*

Initial clinical results obtained with the hepatobiliary contrast agent manganese-DPDP are now available[19,20]. Tumour/liver contrast is significantly higher on T1 weighted images after intravenous application of Mn-DPDP than on non-enhanced images. The improved contrast not only permits the identification of liver metastases as small as 5 mm and thus increases the total number of metastases detected compared with non-enhanced imaging, but also leads to a considerably better demarcation of metastases from surrounding liver tissue[20] (Figure 9.3). Differences in the efficiency of this contrast agent relative to the magnetic field strength have not been reported so far. Another advantage of hepatobiliary contrast material over superparamagnetic iron oxide particles is the fact that it can be used in combination with T1 weighted sequences, which have a higher signal-to-noise ratio and thus yield a better anatomical resolution than T2 weighted images. While liver metastases do not take up hepatobiliary contrast material, hepatogenous tumours do show contrast uptake. The letter include hepatocellular carcinoma, focal nodular hyperplasia and regenerative nodules. This phenomenon, which is well known in nuclear medicine, may open new paths for the differentiation of liver tumours by MR imaging.

### *References*


1. Reinig JW, Dwyer AJ, Miller DK, Frank JA, Adams GW, Chang AE. Liver metastases: detection with MR imaging at 0.5 and 1.5 T. Radiology. 1989;170:149–53.
2. Rummeny EJ, Wernecke K, Saini S, et al. Comparison between high-field-strength MR imaging and CT for screening of hepatic metastases: a receiver operating characteristic analysis. Radiology. 1992;182:879–86.
3. Stark DD, Wittenberg J, Butch RJ, Ferrucci JT. Hepatic metastases: randomized, controlled comparison of detection with MR imaging and CT. Radiology. 1987;165:399–406.
4. Heiken JP, Weyman PJ, Lee JKT, et al. Detection of focal hepatic masses: prospective evaluation with CT, delayed CT, CT during arterial portography, and MR imaging. Radiology. 1989;171:47–51.
5. Li KC, Glazer GM, Quint LE, et al. Distinction of hepatic cavernous hemangioma from hepatic metastases with MR imaging. Radiology. 1988;169:409–415.
6. Rummeny EJ, Weissleder R, Stark DD, et al. Primary liver tumors: diagnosis by MR imaging. AJR. 1989;152:63–72.
7. Wittenberg J, Stark DD, Forman BH, et al. Differentiation of hepatic metastases from hepatic hemangiomas and cysts by using MR imaging. AJR. 1988;151:79–84.
8. Lombardo DM, Baker ME, Spritzer CE, Blinder R, Meyers W, Herfkens RJ. Hepatic hemangiomas vs metastases: MR differentiation at 1.5 T. AJR. 1990;155:55–9.
9. Hamm B, Wolf K-J, Felix R. Conventional and rapid MR imaging of the liver with gadolinium-DTPA. Radiology. 1987;164:313–20.
10. Hamm B, Fischer E, Taupitz M. Differentiation of hepatic hemangiomas from hepatic metastases by using dynamic contrast-enhanced MR imaging. JCAT. 1990;14:205–16.
11. Ohtomo K, Itai Y, Yoshikawa K, et al. Hepatic tumors: dynamic MR imaging. Radiology. 1987;163:27–31.
12. van Beers B, Demeure R, Pringot J, et al. Dynamic spin-echo imaging with Gd-DTPA: value in the differentiation of hepatic tumours. AJR. 1990;154:515–9.
13. Yoshida H, Itai Y, Ohtomo K, Kokubo T, Minami M, Yashiro N. Small hepatocellular carcinoma and cavernous hemangioma: differentiation with dynamic FLASH MR imaging with Gd-DTPA. Radiology. 1989;171:339–42.
14. Mahfouz AE, Hamm B, Taupitz M, Wolf K-J. Hypervascular liver lesions: differentiation of focal nodular hyperplasia from malignant tumors with dynamic gadolinium-enhanced MR imaging. Radiology. 1993;186:133–8.
15. Hamm B, Thoeni RL, Gould B, et al. Comparison of plain and dynamic contrast-enhanced MR imaging in the differentiation of focal liver lesions: a ROC analysis. Radiology. 1992;(P):185.
16. Marchal G, Van Hecke P, Demaerel P, et al. Detection of liver metastases with superparamagnetic iron oxide in 15 patients: results of MR imaging. AJR. 1989;152:771–5.
17. Stark DD, Weissleder R, Elizondo G, et al. Superparamagnetic iron oxide: clinical application as a contrast agent for MR imaging of the liver. Radiology. 1988;186:297–301.
18. Hamm B, Reichel M, Vogl TJ, Taupitz M, Wolf K-J. MR imaging using superparamagnetic iron oxide: clinical results in patients with liver metastases. ROFO.1994;160:52–8.
19. Bernardino ME, Young SW, Lee JKT, Weinreb JC. Hepatic MR imaging with Mn-DPDP: safety, image, quality, and sensitivity. Radiology. 1992;183:53–8.
20. Hamm B, Vogl TJ, Branding G, et al. Focal liver lesions: MR imaging with Mn-DPDP – initial clinical results in 40 patients. Radiology. 1992;182:167–74.

10

# FUTURE TECHNIQUES IN MR IMAGING OF THE LIVER: ECHO PLANAR IMAGING

JOCHEN GAA AND SANJAY SAINI

The dramatic success which magnetic resonance (MR) imaging has achieved in the diagnosis of diseases of the central nervous system has not been mirrored in abdominal applications. Problems associated with MR imaging of the abdomen arise almost entirely because of the artifacts secondary to gross physiological motion (e.g. respiration, peristalsis, cardiac pulsation). In addition, lack of a suitable contrast agent for marking the bowel, and inferior spatial resolution in comparison with computed tomography has limited the use of MR imaging in the abdomen. Recent introduction of fast gradient-echo techniques (scan time approximately 1 s) and echo planar MR (EP-MR) imaging (scan time <100 ms) has allowed radiologists to acquire motion artifact-free MR images[1,2]. In this chapter, we shall review the potential utility of fast imaging techniques, particularly EP-MR imaging in evaluation of the liver.

## Background

The concept of EP-MR imaging was first advanced by Mansfield in 1977[3]. Initial clinical images were obtained in 1983[4] at a field strength of 0.15 T with imaging times of approximately 35 ms. However, interest in echo-planar imaging (EPI) was tempered because images had poor signal-to-noise ratios, low in-plane resolution ($32 \times 32$ matrix), and only infants or young children could be imaged because of a small magnet bore. In 1986, Rzedzian and Pykett developed a prototype adult-sized whole body 2.0 T MR imaging system, with which high-resolution EP-MR images of the heart and abdomen were obtained with the Instascan technique[5–7]. Recent technical advances have resulted in the implementation of echo planar capabilities as an add-on feature on conventional MR systems[2].

## Principles of EP-MR technique

In contrast to conventional pulse sequences, where the total number of excitations equals the number of the desired phase encoding steps (typically 128–256), at EP-MR imaging, the spatial information necessary to generate an image is acquired after

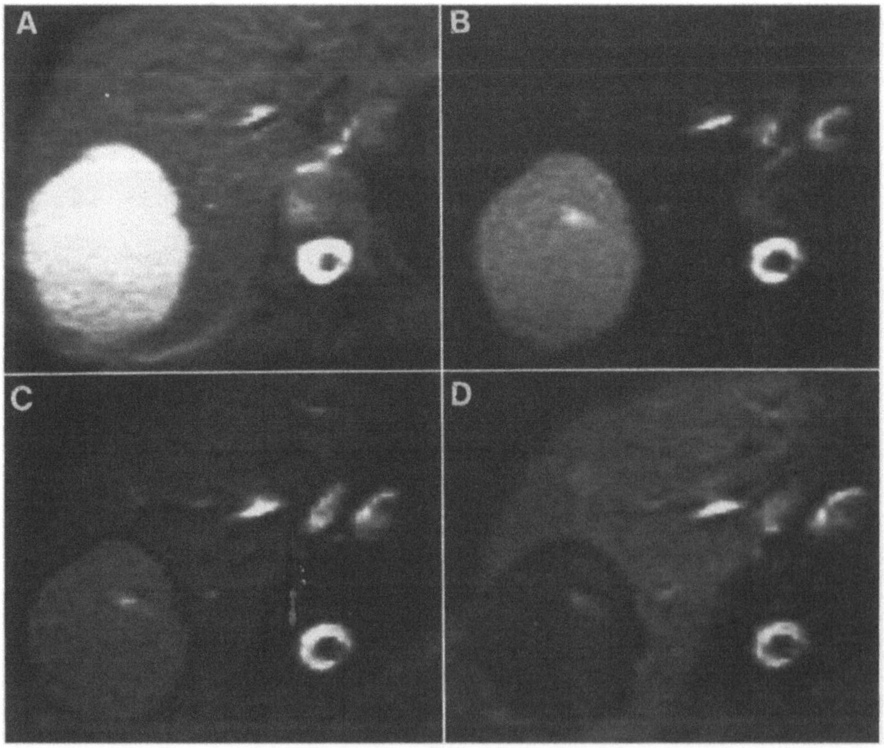


**Figure 10.1** Hemangioma. T1-weighted inversion recovery EP-MR images with TR = infinite, TE = 25 msec, TI = 100 (**A**), 380 (**B**), 600 (**C**), and 800 (**D**) msec. Liver sig' al nulls at 380 (B) while lesion incompletely nulls at TI 800 (D). Low signal intensity rim seen at TI 600 (C) represents voxels at null poi . (Reprinted with permission from reference 14).

a single excitation and images may be acquired in under 100 ms (of course this period is longer for long TE and/or long inversion time (TI) acquisition). However, EP-MR imaging requires specialized costly hardware for fast gradient switching, large peak amplitudes, and fast data acquisition. For a more detailed description of the EP-MR imaging technique, the reader is referred to a review article by Cohen and Weisskoff[2].

Soft-tissue contrast in EP-MR imaging is much like that of conventional MR imaging, making predictions of contrast straightforward. For example, since EP-MR imaging uses only a single excitation pulse it is possible to obtain 'infinite TR' images with a spin echo (SE) pulse sequence. Hence, contrast in T2 weighted SE images is independent of T1 information. Depending on the TE employed, the degree of T2 weighting of the image can be varied. With relatively short TE, the images are predominantly proton density weighted, whereas at longer TE (TE>T2), pure T2 weighted images can be achieved. T2* weighted images can be obtained with the use of gradient echo pulse sequence. T1 weighted contrast is obtained with an inversion recovery (IR) pulse sequence through the use of a preparatory 180° inversion pulse at the beginning of the pulse sequence. In order to eliminate chemical shift artifacts which are more severe at EP-MR imaging, fat suppression is employed on EP-MR images with a frequency selective pulse. Thus, on EP-MR images, fatty tissues, such as subcutaneous and retroperitoneal fat, are dark and abdominal viscera, such as liver, spleen, muscle, intervertebral discs, and fluid-filled bowel, are bright, resulting in increased contrast-to-noise and improved conspicuity for tissue pathology[8].

## Instascan EP-MR imaging technique

Our abdominal EP-MR imaging experience based on scanning is performed with the Instascan (Advanced NMR Systems, Wilmington, MA) technique on a modified 1.5T Sigma scanner (General Electric Medical Systems, Milwaukee, W1)[2]. Fat-suppressed axial 10-mm contiguous slices are obtained to cover the liver (up to 21 slices). A single 12-second breath-

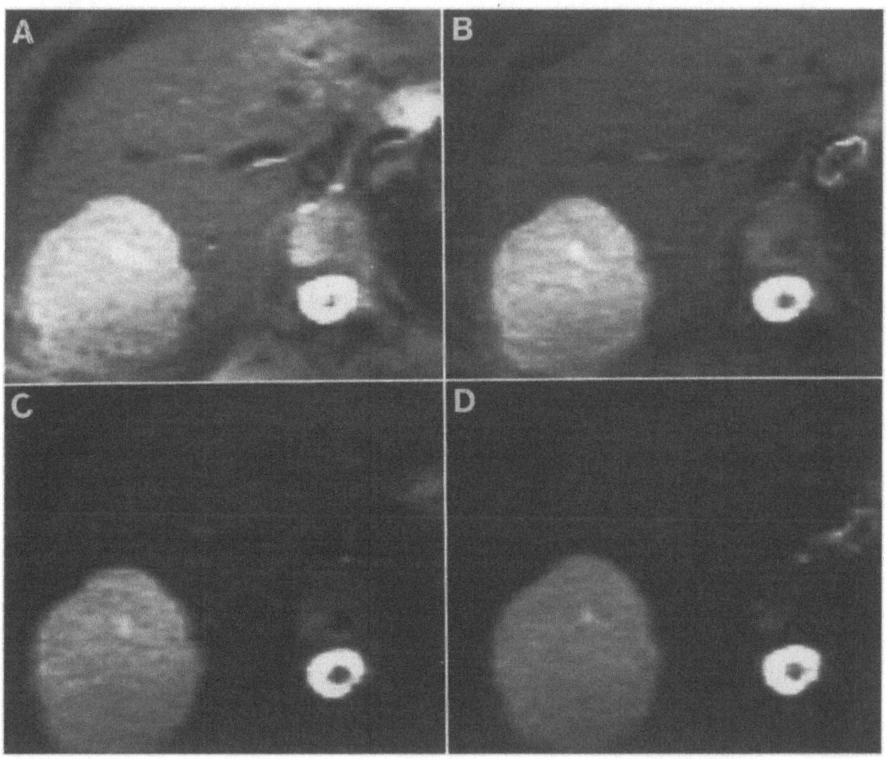


**Figure 10.2** Hemangioma. T2-weighted SE EP-MR images: TR = infinite, TE = 25 (**A**), 50 (**B**), 100 (**C**), and 150 (**D**) msec. Liver with short T2 shows signal loss at longer TEs in comparison to hemangioma which remains bright because of its longer T2.

hold is necessary to eliminate effects of cross-talk. As noted before T1 and T2 weighted images are obtained by using inversion recovery (IR) and spin echo pulse sequences (SE), respectively. T1 weighted images with infinite TR are acquired at a TE of 20 ms (minimum) with T1 of 380 ms (to null liver), and 600–1000 ms (to null lesions) (Figures 10.1 and 10.3). T2 weighted images with infinite TR are acquired at TEs of 25, 50, 100 and 150 ms (Figures 10.2 and 10.4). A matrix size of 128 × 128 with either a 20 (phase) × 40 (frequency) cm (normal subjects) or a 40 × 40 cm (large patients) field-of-view (FOV) is used. This results in an in-plane resolution of 1.5 mm (phase) × 3.0 mm (frequency) or 3.0 mm × 3.0 mm for the larger FOV. High MR resolution images using EP techniques require >1 excitation. Hence, TR can no longer be infinite, which introduces T1 contamination in T2 weighted images. In addition, the duration of the breath hold becomes unacceptably long for abdominal imaging.

## Clinical applications

The two major goals of MR imaging of the liver are cancer detection and lesional tissue characterization[9]. In the discussion that follows, we shall address each of these aspects separately.

For liver lesion detection, the performance of EP-MR imaging has not been investigated rigorously. On theoretical grounds, it is expected that EP-MR imaging might show better performance than conventional MR for detection of lesions located in the left lobe of the liver because these single-shot images freeze physiological motion from cardiac pulsation. Similarly, these images will be superior in unco-operative patients. Furthermore, the high soft-tissue contrast in purely T2 weighted EP-MR images might be of advantage in lesion conspicuity. Additionally, the feasibility of rapid EP-MR angiography can allow distinction between vessels and lesions. However, due to large biological variation in relaxation times of liver and liver tumours, native

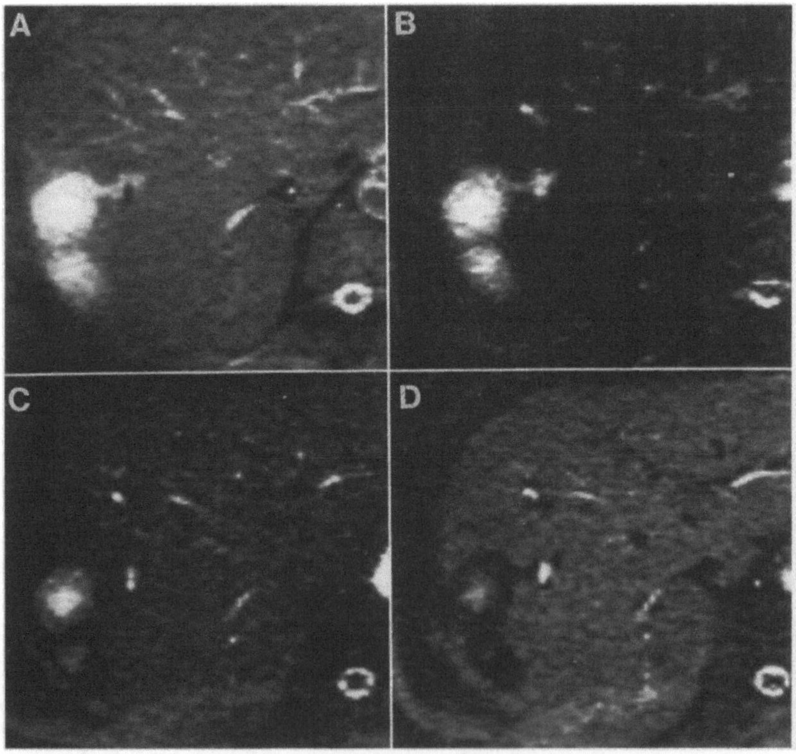


**Figure 10.3** Metastases. T1-weighted inversion recovery EP-MR images with TR = infinite, TE = 25 msec, TI = 100 (**A**), 380 (**B**), 600 (**C**), and 800 (**D**) msec. Liver signal nulls at TI 380 (B) while rim of metastases nulls at TI 800 (D). The central cystic area would have nulled at a longer TI.

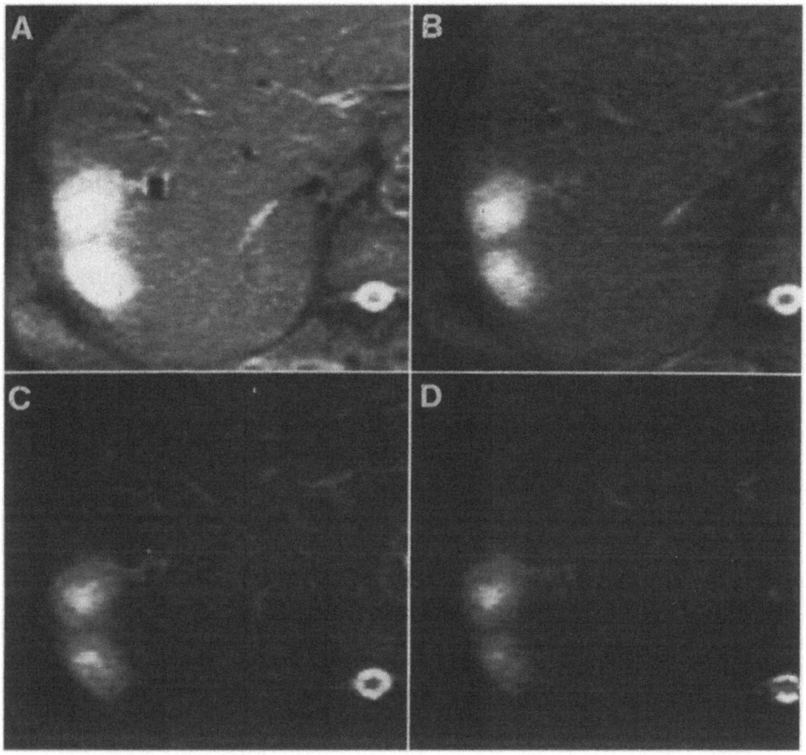

**Figure 10.4** Metastases. T2-weighted SE EP-MR images: TR = infinite, TE = 25 (**A**), 50 (**B**), 100 (**C**), and 150 (**D**) msec. Lesions are hyperintense with respect to liver but less intense than CSF.

soft-tissue contrast is not likely to be sufficient for lesion detection. Therefore tissue-specific MR contrast agents will still be needed to improve lesion conspicuity. Another disadvantage of the present system is the 20 × 40 cm field of view necessary for providing in-plane resolution comparable to conventional MR images. In many patients, this results in wrap-around artifacts and in incomplete evaluation of the liver. On the other hand, short examination times (e.g. 4 breath-holds in less than 5 minutes) can increase throughput of patients screened for possible hepatic metastases.

Liver lesion characterization is important because autopsy studies have shown a high prevalence (>20%) of benign hepatic tumours in an adult population[10]. For the purpose of tissue characterization by MR imaging, various qualitative and quantitative parameters have been proposed and the importance of T2 weighted images has been emphasized[11–13]. Unfortunately, tissue characterization with conventional MR imaging has been difficult, particularly at high field strength, because of overlap in the qualitative characterization and the image-derived quantitative measurements of solid and non-solid lesions. As reported recently, EP-MR imaging is useful for characterizing focal hepatic lesions using T2 calculations[14]. For classifying lesions as solid (non-cysts and non-haemangiomas) or non-solid (cysts and haemangiomas) a T2 cutoff of 116 ms was 100% accurate for classifying lesions as solid or non-solid and 93% accurate for characterizing them as benign or malignant (Figure 10.5). This high accuracy of EP-MR imaging in lesion characterization is believed to be due to the absence of motion-induced volume averaging and phase artifacts, the ability to obtain purely T2 weighted images, and the use of multiple data points to calculate T2 relaxation times. As reported, these considerations are particularly relevant in characterization of small (<2 cm in size) liver lesions. The use of gadolinium-chelates to evaluate liver lesion perfusion for tissue characterization is not likely to be of any greater advantage at EP-MR imaging than with conventional MR imaging. The principal reason for this is that liver lesion perfusion occurs over a period

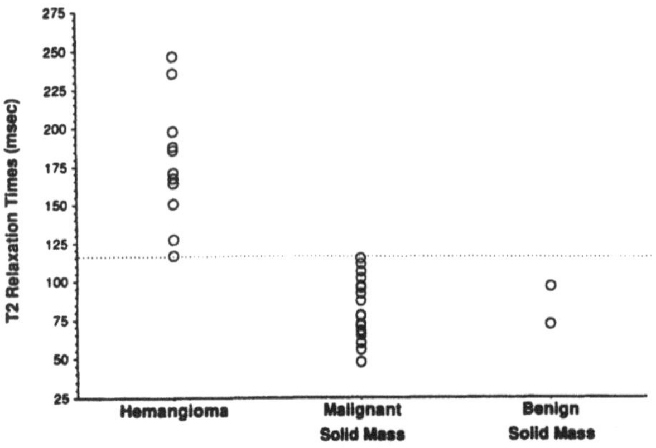


**Figure 10.5** Scattergram of lesion T2 times. Note clear separation between haemangiomas and solid lesions. This was not present on a T1 scattergram (not shown). (Reprinted with permission from Reference 14)

of seconds and faster scanning is not necessary. Hence, fast gradient-echo techniques are adequate to allow demonstration of tumour perfusion. In addition, at EP-MR imaging, T1 weighting is obtained with an IR pulse sequence and gadolinium-enhanced dynamic scanning is performed using a T1 which nulls the tissue (lesion). This creates several problems at dynamic imaging, including non-availability of long TR (necessary for IR pulse sequences) and a complex response of tissue SI to gadolinium-related proton-relaxation enhancement. The latter effect produces signal loss in structures having comparatively longer T1 times (T1 shortening brings them closer to the null point) and signal increase in structures with shorter T1 times (T1 shortening takes them further away from the null point).

## Conclusion

Several fast imaging techniques (e.g. Multisection FLASH, RASE, EP-MR) have been developed to examine the liver in a single 12–25-second breath-hold[2,15,16]. Hence, fundamentally these techniques are similar although EP-MR images will be less sensitive to motion artifacts if the patient breathes during the scan because the period of data acquisition for each image is an order of magnitude less (100 ms versus 1–25 s)[8]. In addition, the higher soft tissue contrast or purely T2 weighted images without residual T1 contamination might be helpful for liver lesion detection although tissue-specific contrast agents will still be needed to overcome inherent limitations in intrinsic soft-tissue contrast. The short scan time will also permit implementation of a time-efficient integrated MR examination which can include T1 weighted, T2 weighted, MR angiographic and dynamic MR imaging. This will be of benefit in the examination of unco-operative patients and might result in increased patient throughput.

### *References*


1. Chien D, Edelman RR. Fast magnetic resonance imaging. In: Higgins CB, Hricak H, Helms CA, eds. Magnetic resonance imaging of the body. New York: Raven Press; 1992:175–98.
2. Cohen MS, Weisskoff RM. Ultra-fast imaging. Magn Reson Imaging. 1991:9:1–37.
3. Mansfield P. Multi-planar image formation using NMR spin echoes. J Phys. 1977:C10:L55–L58.
4. Rzedzian RR. Mansfield P. Doyle M, et al. Real-time NMR clinical imaging in pediatrics. Lancet. 1983;2:1281–2.
5. Rzedzian RR, Pykett IL. An instant scan technique for real-time MR imaging (abstr). Radiology. 1986;161(P):333.
6. Rzedzian RR, Pykett IL. Instant images of the human heart using a new, whole body MR imaging system. AJR. 1987; 149:245–50.
7. Pykett IL, Rzedzian RR. Instant images of the body by magnetic resonance. Magn Reson Med. 1987;5:563–571.
8. Saini S, Stark DD, Rzedzian RR, et al. Forty-millisecond MR imaging of the abdomen at 2.0 T. Radiology. 1989; 173:111–6.
9. Ferrucci JT. Liver tumour imaging: current concepts. AJR. 1990;155:473–84.
10. Karhunen PJ. Benign hepatic tumors and tumor like conditions in men. J Clin Pathol. 1986;39:183–8.
11. Wittenberg J, Stark DD, Forman BH, et al. Differentiation of hepatic metastases from hepatic hemangiomas and cysts. AJR. 1988;151:79–84.
12. Egglin TK, Rummeny E, Stark DD, Wittenberg J, Saini S, Ferrucci JT. Hepatic tumors: quantitative tissue characterization with MR imaging. Radiology. 1990;176:107–10.
13. Lombardo DM, Baker ME, Spritzer CE, Blinder R, Meyers W, Herfkens RJ. Hepatic hemangiomas vs metastases: MR differentiation at 1.5 T, AJR. 1990;155:55–9.
14. Goldberg MA, Hahn PF, Saini S, et al. Values of T1 and T2 relaxation times from echoplanar MR imaging in the characterization of focal hepatic lesions. AJR. 1993;160:1011–7.
15. Mirowitz SA, Lee JKT, Brown JJ, Eilenberg SS, Heiken JP, Perman WM. Rapid acquisition spin-echo (RASE) MR imaging: a new technique for reduction of artifacts and acquisition time. Radiology. 1990;175:131–5.
16. Taupitz M, Hamm B, Speidel A, Deimling M, Branding G, Wolf KJ. Multisection FLASH: method for breath-hold MR imaging of the entire liver. Radiology. 1992;183:73–9.

# INDEX

# SERIES IN RADIOLOGY

1. J.O. Op den Orth: *The Standard Biphasic-contrast Examination of the Stomach and Duodenum.* Method, Results, and Radiological Atlas. 1979 ISBN 90-247-2159-8
2. J.L. Sellink and R.E. Miller: *Radiology of the Small Bowel.* Modern Enteroclysis Technique and Atlas. 1982 ISBN 90-247-2460-0
3. R.E. Miller and J. Skucas: *The Radiological Examination of the Colon.* Practical Diagnosis. 1983 ISBN 90-247-2666-2
4. S. Forgács: *Bones and Joints in Diabetes Mellitus.* 1982 ISBN 90-247-2395-7
5. Gy. Németh and H. Kuttig (eds.): *Isodose Atlas for Use in Radiotherapy.* 1981 ISBN 90-247-2476-7
6. J. Chermet: *Atlas of Phlebography of the Lower Limbs.* Including the Iliac Veins. 1982 ISBN 90-247-2525-9
7. B.K. Janevski: *Angiography of the Upper Extremity.* 1982 ISBN 90-247-2684-0
8. M.A.M. Feldberg: *Computed Tomography of the Retroperitoneum.* An Anatomical and Pathological Atlas with Emphasis on the Fascial Planes. 1983 ISBN 0-89838-573-3
9. L.E.H. Lampmann, S.A. Duursma and J.H.J. Ruys: *CT Densitometry in Osteoporosis.* The Impact on Management of the Patient. 1984 ISBN 0-89838-633-0
10. J.J. Broerse and T.J. Macvittie: *Response of Different Species to Total Body Irradiation.* 1984 ISBN 0-89838-678-0
11. C. L'Herminé: *Radiology of Liver Circulation.* 1985 ISBN 0-89838-715-9
12. G. Maatman: *High-resolution Computed Tomography of the Paranasal Sinuses, Pharynx and Related Regions.* Impact of CT Identification on Diagnosis and Patient Management. 1986 ISBN 0-89838-802-3
13. C. Plets, A.L. Baert, G.L. Nijs and G. Wilms: *Computer Tomographic Imaging and Anatomic Correlation of the Human Brain.* A Comparative Atlas of Thin CT-scan Sections and Correlated Neuro-anatomic Preparations. 1987 ISBN 0-89838-811-2
14. J. Valk: *MRI of the Brain, Head, Neck and Spine.* A Teaching Atlas of Clinical Applications. 1987 ISBN 0-89838-957-7
15. J.L. Sellink: *X-Ray Differential Diagnosis in Small Bowel Disease.* A Practical Approach. 1988 ISBN 0-89838-351-X
16. Th.H.M. Falke (ed.): *Essentials of Clinical MRI.* 1988 ISBN 0-89838-353-6
17. B.D. Fornage: *Endosonography.* 1989 ISBN 0-7923-0047-5
18. R. Chisin (ed.): *MRI/CT and Pathology in Head and Neck Tumors.* A Correlative Study. 1989 ISBN 0-7923-0227-3
19. G. Gozzetti, A. Mazziotti, L. Bolondi and L. Barbara (eds.): *Intraoperative Ultrasonography in Hepato-biliary and Pancreatic Surgery.* A Practical Guide. With Contributions by Y. Chapuis, J.-F. Gigot and P.-J. Kestens. 1989 ISBN 0-7923-0261-3
20. A.M.A. De Schepper and H.R.M. Degryse: *Magnetic Resonance Imaging of Bone and Soft Tissue Tumors and Their Mimics.* A Clinical Atlas. With Contributions by F. De Belder, L. van den Houwe, F. Ramon, P. Parizel and N. Buyssens. 1989 ISBN 0-7923-0343-1
21. J.O. Barentsz, F.M.J. Debruyne and S.H.J. Ruijs: *Magnetic Resonance Imaging of Carcinoma of the Urinary Bladder.* With a Forword by H. Hricak and R. Hohenfellner. 1990 ISBN 0-7923-0838-7
22. C. Depré, J.A. Melin, W. Wijns, R. Demeure, F. Hammer and J. Pringot: *Atlas of Cardiac MR Imaging with Anatomical Correlations.* Foreword by Alexander R. Margulis. 1991 ISBN 0-7923-0941-3
23. J.A. Castelijns, G.B. Snow and J. Valk: *MR Imaging of Laryngeal Cancer.* With Contributions by G.J. Gerritsen and W.N. Hanafee. 1991 ISBN 0-7923-1101-9
24. R.H. Mohiaddin and D.B. Longmore: *MRI Atlas of Normal Anatomy.* 1992 ISBN 0-7923-8974-3
25. B. Hamm, H-P. Niendorf and Th. Balzer (eds.): *Contrast Agents in Liver Imaging.* 1994 ISBN 0-7923-3130-3

KLUWER ACADEMIC PUBLISHERS – DORDRECHT / BOSTON / LONDON

MIX
Papier aus verantwortungsvollen Quellen
Paper from responsible sources
FSC® C105338

If you have any concerns about our products,
you can contact us on
**ProductSafety@springernature.com**

In case Publisher is established outside the EU,
the EU authorized representative is:
**Springer Nature Customer Service Center GmbH**
**Europaplatz 3, 69115 Heidelberg, Germany**

Printed by Libri Plureos GmbH
in Hamburg, Germany